To Céleste and her Mom and Dad

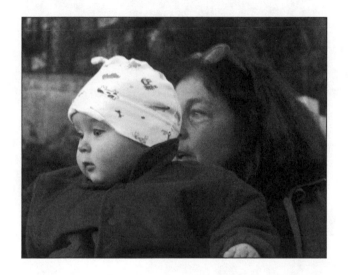

The secret of a better world
lives in the hearts of our children

With Gratitude to my Yoga Masters,

Baba Muktananda
and
Gurumayi Chidvilasananda

Playful
FAMILY YOGA
For Kids, Parents and Grandparents

Teressa Asencia

Elysian Editions
Princeton Book Company, Publishers

Although the author has made every effort to ensure that the poses presented in this book are safe for home practice, please listen to your body and practice only the poses that are comfortable for you. If you have any health problems or any doubt about which poses are suitable for you, please consult with your doctor or health care practitioner before practicing these Yoga poses. The author, publisher, participants and distributors of this book disclaim any liability in connection with the exercises and advice herein.

Elysian Editions
Princeton Book Company, Publishers
P.O. Box 831
Hightstown, NJ 08520-0831

Photographs by Wes Gerrish, Teressa Asencia,
Cheng Kun Lin, Tracy Bennett and Joshua Nachman

Book design and composition by Lisa Denham

Library of Congress Cataloging–in–Publication Data
Asencia, Teressa
    Playful family yoga for kids, parents and grandparents/ Teressa Asencia
        p. cm.
        Summary: Presents a yoga routine that guides children, using pictures and words, into poses with friends and family members.
        ISBN 0-87127-252-0
        1. Yoga, Hatha, for children–Juvenile literature. [1. Yoga] I.Title.
    RA781.7 .A82 2002
    613.7'046'083–dc21

                                                                2002035054

Printed in the US   5 4 3 2 1

Contents

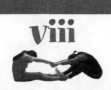

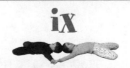

Introduction

There is a saying in the ancient Yoga scriptures: "If the body is weak, if the veins and nerves are weak, if there is no strength in the life force, then how can we derive any joy from living?" People everywhere are realizing that the foundation of happiness is health. The stress of today's world causes us to yearn for ancient, yet simple, Yoga techniques that nourish the body, refresh the mind and create a feeling of unity among all people.

The science of Yoga was developed five thousand years ago when ancient sages spontaneously went into Yoga positions during meditation. The word Yoga means "yoke" or union. It is the art of uniting the individual soul with the universal soul. This ancient art involves a series of physical exercises and breathing techniques designed to rejuvenate every part of the body and calm the mind. It is one of the most comprehensive forms of physical exercise for people of all ages.

While relaxing the body, rejuvenating the internal organs, and calming the mind, Yoga postures also tone the muscles, soothe the nervous system, and energize the body. Certain poses improve digestion, enhance circulation and regulate the glandular system. Others enhance endurance, inspire moral courage and strengthen the spirit; and, as apparent in this book, bring joy.

Yoga is beneficial for children and is becoming popular in education. Some schools have already trained teachers to include Yoga as a regular part of the classroom day. It helps students concentrate and release tension, especially when they are under stress.

Traditionally, Yoga has been a solitary practice. *Playful Family Yoga* presents a new, creative form of Yoga designed to practice with a partner. This unique book describes how children and their families can enjoy practicing Yoga. The captivating, playful photographs depict the joy inherent in this fun and creative form of Yoga.

This innovative approach to the ancient art of Yoga allows two people to use the support and counterbalance to go deeper into the poses than is possible when practicing alone. Supported poses are emotionally nourishing and have a powerful psychological effect. They are restful and rejuvenating, and tone the body with minimum effort.

Each of the six chapters in *Playful Family Yoga* presents a complete partner Yoga routine. Although the photographs in each chapter depict specific ages and relationships, the routines are universal and may be practiced by people of all ages. This practical approach of incorporating ancient Yoga techniques into modern daily life will enable families, children, couples and people of all ages to spend time with their loved ones renewing body, mind and spirit.

Author's Note

Many years ago, when I took my first Yoga class to get back in shape after the birth of my son, I discovered that Yoga was much more than just physical exercise. Through regular Yoga practice, I experienced that in addition to helping me stay in shape, Yoga enhanced my health and made me feel great. Since then, Yoga has continued to spontaneously expand in my life.

During the past twenty-five years, I have lived in many countries where I was blessed with the opportunity to share my enjoyment of Yoga with people from many cultures. This book expresses my appreciation and gratitude to my students and friends around the world whose photos so beautifully demonstrate that the joy of Yoga may be enjoyed by anyone, anytime, in any place.

May it encourage people of all ages to improve their health as they enhance their relationships, bringing more love and joy into their daily lives. May it inspire people in all parts of the world to experience the unity inherent in all creation.

Advice for Home Practice

Please remember to wait two hours after eating before practicing Yoga. Listen to your body and never strain. The secret of Yoga is to concentrate on the breath, allowing the body to relax more with each exhalation. Pregnant women should consult with their doctor or a teacher who specializes in prenatal Yoga and should never practice any poses that put strain on the abdomen. Women who are menstruating should not practice inverted poses. When practicing with a partner, always respect each other's limits.

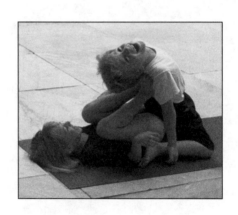

Chapter One
Friendship Poses

When we are happy
love radiates from us like light from the sun

With an eye made quiet by the power of harmony and the deep power of joy, we see into the life of things.
—William Wordsworth

This series of supporting and counterbalancing poses for two is designed to uncover the joy that is our true nature. Inherent in all the Yoga poses is the rasa or nectar that the pose reveals. This delightful series of stretching exercises and invigorating postures is designed to develop flexibility, strength and concentration as it inspires deeper friendship and transports us into the wellspring of joy that is always inside us.

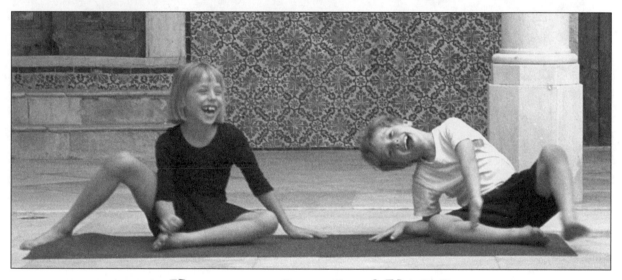

Have you heard of Yoga?
"Mom said you have to be a pretzel to do yoga."
"I like pretzels. Let's try it!"

1

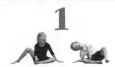

Sailboat Stretch

Sit facing your partner with your legs open wide. Put the bottoms of your feet together and hold your partner's left hand.

Now, open your sails by stretching your right arm toward the back. Gently, pull away from your partner and look back at your right hand. Good!

Close your eyes and imagine you are sailing through a big blue ocean.

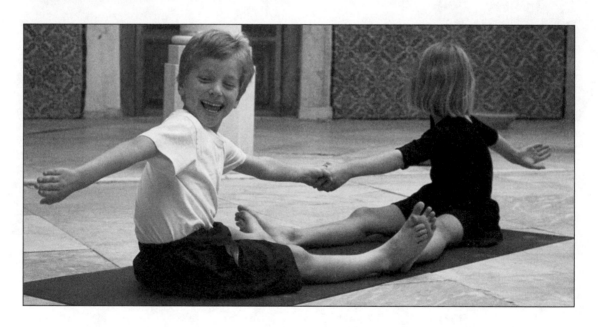

"This feels great!"

"Do you feel the wind in your sails?"

Partner Pigeon

BENEFITS: The Pigeon Pose is a classic Yoga pose for opening the hips. The polarity created by pressing against your partner's palms creates a deeper opening in the hip joints, allowing you to go further into the pose than you could on your own. This pose also expands the spine and strenghtens the arms.

Sit facing your partner. Bend one knee and stretch the other leg straight back. Now turn your torso to face your partner and place the palms of your hands together. Gently press against your partner's hands.

Imagine that you have roots that go deep into the earth. Inhaling, breathe into your chest and expand up through your spine. Great!

How do you feel?

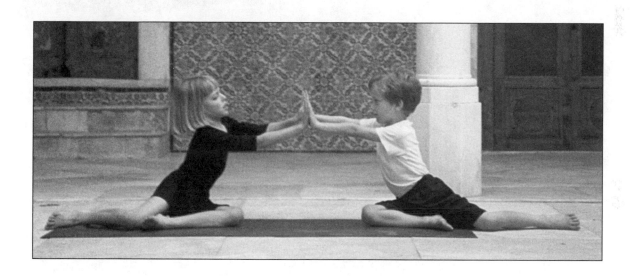

"I feel like a plant that's growing fast. "

"I feel like a happy pigeon!"

Boat Pose

Sit facing your partner with your legs open a few inches and place the soles of your feet together. Now, gently press your feet against your partner's and slowly raise your legs together at the same time.

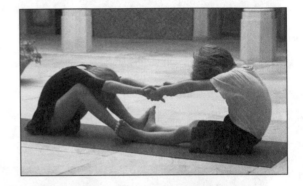

Stretch up through the spine as you continue to press your feet and pull gently against your partner's hands to keep your balance. Bravo!

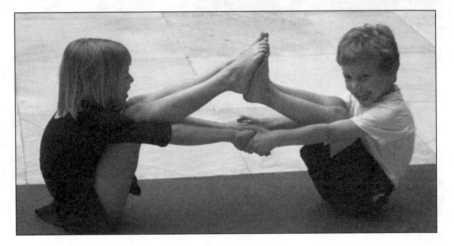

"I can't do that."

"Yes you can."

"Just push my feet exactly the same as I push yours!"

4

Boat Pose

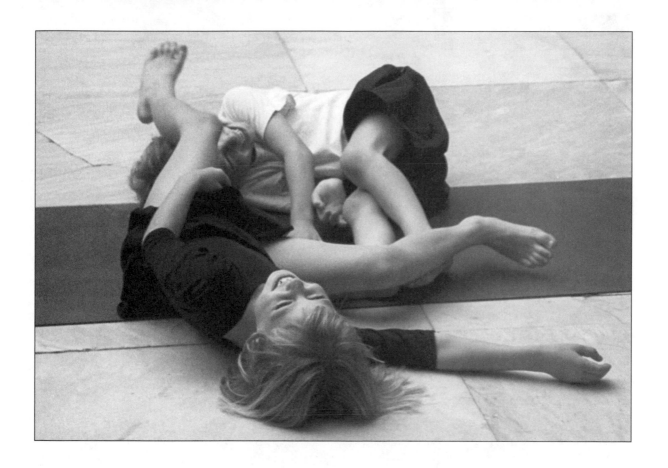

"We did it!"

"That was fun!"

Table Pose

Partner One, come up on your hands and knees, then sit back on your heels and bring your forehead to the floor. Rest here with the palms of your hands on the floor near your head. This position is called the Child's Pose which will be the base for many other poses.

Partner Two, gently sit down on your partner, placing your tailbone on top of his. Now lie back to rest your back on your partner's back. Breathe in deeply as you reach your arms overhead and place one hand on top of the other with the palms facing the sky. Exhale slowly as you stretch your legs long and place the bottoms of your feet on the floor.

Rest here, breathing in deeply and breathing out long, several times.

How do you feel?

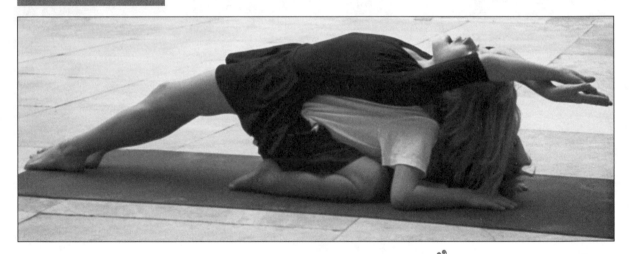

"My body is still as a mountain."

"My breath is flowing like a river."

Camel Pose

BENEFITS: The Camel Pose is a traditional Yoga pose that tones the liver, pancreas and kidneys. Practicing the partner version of this pose strengthens the legs and the abdominal muscles of the partner on the floor and allows the partner on top to expand the chest and shoulders with minimum effort. It improves posture and gives a massage to the shoulder blades and upper back, creating a wonderful release in the heart chakra in the center of the chest.

Partner One, lie on your back and bend your knees into your chest.

Partner Two, kneel in front of your partner, placing your feet alongside her hips. Carefully, relax back against her feet.

With each inhalation, breathe into your chest as your partner gently presses her feet into your back, allowing you to expand more.

Close your eyes and imagine you are riding through the desert on a huge camel.

What's the difference between a camel and a dromedary?

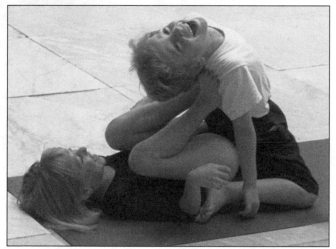

"A camel has two humps and a dromedary has one."
"Maybe this should be called
the dromedary pose!"

7

Starship

BENEFITS: The Starship Pose opens the shoulder joints, stretches the arms and creates a feeling of partnership.

Begin by sitting side by side with the inside leg stretched out in front. Now, bend your outside leg at the knee and place the bottom of your foot on the inside of your thigh.

Bring your inside hands together and stretch your arms forward. At the same time, clasp your hands in back and stretch your back arms toward the back. Continue to breathe in deeply, and stretch up through the top of your head.

Feel how this double stretch of the arms opens the shoulders and allows you to expand up through your spine more.

Close your eyes, continue to breathe deeply and imagine you are growing bigger and bigger.

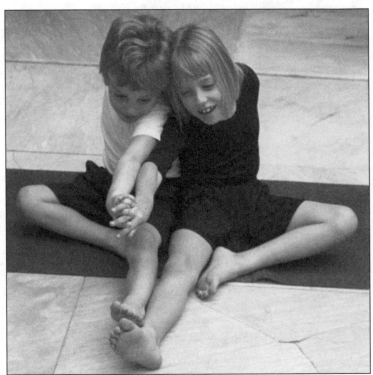

"Do you feel like we're expanding into the universe?"
"Yes. Beam me up, Scotty!"

Two Frogs On A Lotus

BENEFITS: This pose releases the hip joints, opens the shoulder joints and expands the spinal column, creating space between the vertebrae.

Sit in a squatting position opposite your partner. Reach your arms forward to hold hands with your partner. Keep your arms alongside your ears and breathe in deeply. Feel the breath expanding all the way down your spine.

Now, concentrate on the tailbone at the base of your spine and imagine you have a heavy tail. Breathe out long and feel your tail gently move a bit closer to the floor as your arms gently pull against your partner's arms.

Do you feel your hip joints opening and your spine and shoulder joints expanding?

Close your eyes and imagine you are as light as a frog sitting on a lotus flower.

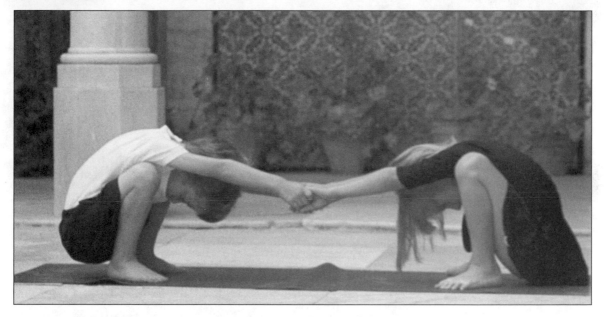

" Let's pretend we're floating on a beautiful lotus leaf in Grandma's pond."

"Ribbit...Ribbit"

London Bridge

Stand opposite your partner. As you breathe out, gently bend forward from the waist and take your partner's hands.

Keep holding your partner's hands and slowly take a few baby steps backward until your arms are straight. Keep your arms alongside your ears as you breathe in. Feel the breath expand down the spine, all the way down the legs and into the feet.

Imagine your legs are strong as steel and feel your spine expanding. Rest here breathing in deeply and breathing out long. With each exhalation, feel the muscles around the shoulders relax.

Do you feel this pose releasing the shoulders, stretching the spine and making your legs strong?

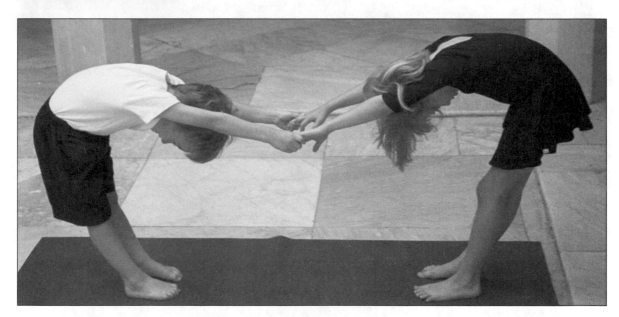

"My legs feel strong as London Bridge!"
"It feels like my arms are growing longer."

Double Dog

Partner One, come up on your hands and knees. Now, push your hands into the floor to straighten both arms and legs and lift up into an upside down V position. Rest here in the Yoga pose called the Downward Dog.

Partner Two, stand with your feet alongside Partner One's hands. Very gently and carefully, sit down on her back, and slowly lie back to rest your back on her back. Relax into the pose, letting your head fall back and your arms release to the sides.

Rest here, breathing together for several breaths. When you are ready to come out of the pose, Partner Two, slowly roll back up to sit on your partner's shoulders and then gently stand up. Partner One, walk your hands toward your feet and then slowly roll up to a standing position.

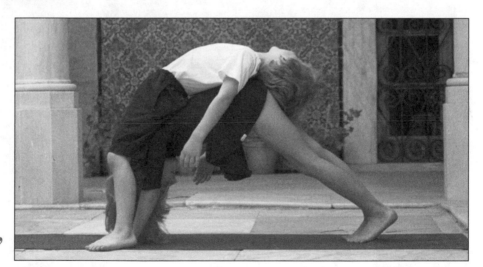

"How do you feel?"

"This feels great!"

"Let's reverse positions and try it with you on top!"

The Bobsled

BENEFITS: This pose expands the chest and opens the shoulder joints. It also releases tension in the neck and shoulders and develops the ability to tune into each other and work together as a team.

Partner One, sit behind your partner and stretch your legs out. Place your left foot on your partner's lower back and your right foot on the center of his back at heart level.

Partner Two, sit with your legs stretched out in front and reach your arms back to hold hands with your partner. Partner One, very gently pull his arms back as you press your feet a bit more into his back, enhancing the stretch.

Rest here, breathing in deeply and breathing out long together. With each inhalation, feel the spine expand. With each exhalation, feel the chest and shoulder joints expand.

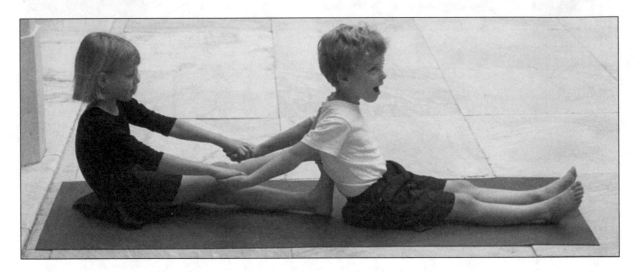

" Let's close our eyes and imagine we're sliding down a big snowy mountain."

"Do you feel the wind and snow in your face?"

Heaven and Earth

Partner One, come up on hands and knees. Partner Two, gently sit down on your partner placing your tailbone on top of his tailbone. Now, slowly lie down on his back and relax your arms to the sides.

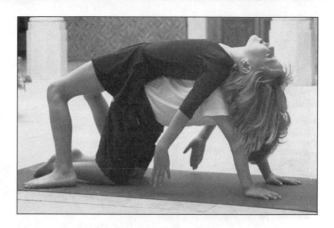

Partner One, push on your hands to round your back, allowing your partner to expand her chest and release her arms more.

On the next inhalation, breathe into your lower back. Feel your lower back expand against your partner's lower back.

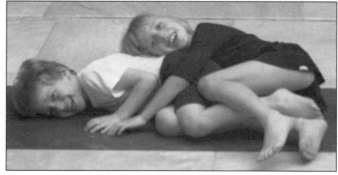

Now, begin to rock slightly. Inhaling, rock back. Exhaling, rock forward. Continue at your own rhythm. Feel how this motion allows the partner on top to relax more.

When you are ready to come out of the pose, Partner One will sit back into the Child's Pose as your partner slowly rolls off.

" That was so relaxing!"

"Let's reverse roles and try it with you on the top!"

The Diamond

Sit facing your partner with your legs spread as wide as possible and the soles of your feet together. Hold your partner's left hand.

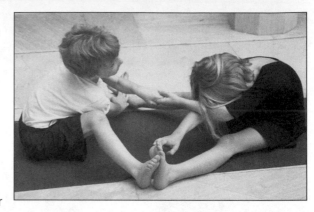

Now, stretch your right arm under your left arm and reach toward your left foot. If it is easy, hold your left foot. If it is difficult for you to reach your left foot, try bending your knees.

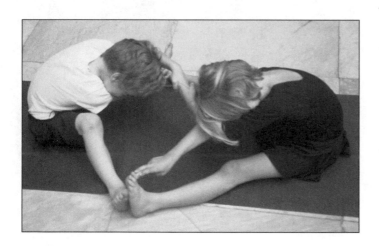

Rest here for three deep breaths. With each inhalation, feel your spinal column expanding. With each exhalation, pull gently on your partner's hand and feel your hip joints relax, allowing you to stretch your right hand a bit more toward your left foot.

At the end of the third exhalation, gently release your foot and expand back up to the center. Close your eyes and look inside your body. Do you feel more expanded inside?

" I feel a space in my hip joints."

"I feel like my spine is longer."

Sleeping Beetle

BENEFITS: This restful pose rejuvenates tired legs and refreshes both body and mind. The reversed blood flow gives a rest to the heart, nourishes the upper body and soothes the nervous system. Concentrating on the space between the eyebrows, sometimes called the third eye, develops our intuition. Practicing this pose together is emotionally nourishing and creates a feeling of harmony and union.

Lie down on your back and scoot up toward your partner until your hips are touching. Now, lift your legs up and let the backs of your legs rest against your partner's legs.

Close your eyes and imagine a window in the space between your eyebrows. Open the window and breathe in deeply. Exhaling, breathe out long. Feel the subtle stream of breath come out the window in the space between the eyebrows. Rest here for several deep breaths and imagine a new way of seeing, with your eyes closed.

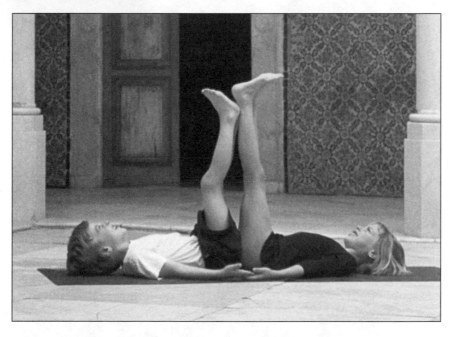

" Mom calls it intuition."
"It feels so good!"

Contemplation

Remember a moment when you
felt completely happy.

Concentrate on that experience
of perfect joy.

Now follow that feeling inside
your own heart.

Experience how joy lives in the
deepest place in the heart.

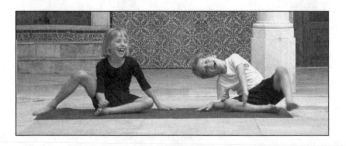

Chapter Two

Yoga Playmates

You may be young, but you are not small.

This series of playful partner poses is designed to give children between the ages of two and twelve an experience of their inner greatness. This creative partner routine will use partner support and counterbalance to open the body, mind and heart. These dynamic, fun partner poses will keep young bodies strong and supple, develop concentration and stimulate the creative abilities innate in every child.

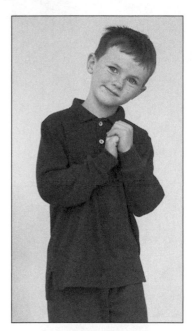

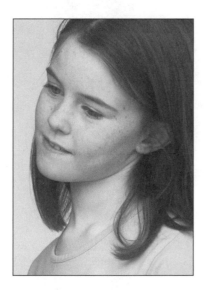

"I don't think I'd like climbing on people!"

"Just try it. You'll like it."

Easy Pose

BENEFITS: This is one of the classic yoga poses that straightens the spine, slows the metabolism and calms the mind.

Sit with your back touching your partner's back and cross your legs. Rest here, breathing with your partner. Inhaling, breathe in deeply, filling your body with breath and energy. Now, exhale together, long and slow. On the next inhalation, imagine the breath coming in the center top of the head and expanding all the way down the spine. Hold the breath in for a moment and concentrate on the base of your spine. Exhaling, visualize the breath expanding up through the spine and out the center top of your head. Continue this deep breathing up and down the spine with your partner for a few minutes. Do you find this pose easy?

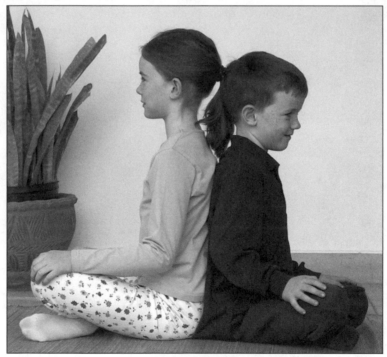

"It's almost too easy."
"Whoever named this pose wasn't kidding."

Spinal Twist

BENEFITS: This simple twist stimulates the thousands of nerve endings in the spine and stimulates the liver. It is a great warm-up pose to prepare the spine for the more advanced poses.

Sit with your back touching your partner's back and your legs crossed. Inhaling, breathe into your lower back and feel it expand against your partner's lower back. Exhaling, twist toward the left, placing your left hand on your partner's right knee. Place your right hand on your own left knee. Rest here for a few breaths, breathing with your partner. With each inhalation, let your spine expand up and feel your lower back and shoulders expanding against your partner's. With each exhalation, gently twist a bit more toward the left.

On the next inhalation, return to center. Exhaling, twist toward the right and place your left hand on your partner's right knee. Place your left hand on your own right knee. Rest here, breathing in deeply and breathing out long with your partner. Again, with each inhalation, feel your lower back and shoulders expand against your partner's. With each exhalation, twist a little bit more toward the right.

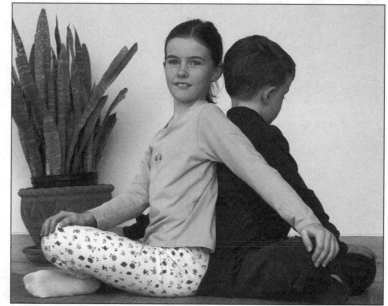

"Do you feel the twist?"

"Especially when I pull against his knee."

"When I pull with both my hands, I can twist more."

19

Touching Toes Together

BENEFITS: This forward bend gives a nice massage to all the abdominal organs. It also stretches the back, elongates the spine and nourishes the thousands of nerve endings in the spinal column.

Sit facing your partner with your legs stretched to the front and the soles of your feet touching. Exhaling, bend forward and try to touch your toes with your fingers. As you rest here, breathing together, try to keep your arms alongside your ears. If it is difficult to touch your toes, bend your knees a little to make it easier to bend forward

As you breathe in deeply, imagine the breath expanding through your body, into your legs and all the way down into your feet. Gently, press your feet against your partner's feet. As you exhale, let your body soften allowing your chest to move more toward your knees.

Rest here a few breaths. Let the breath help you go deeper into the pose. With each inhalation, feel the breath expanding your torso and spine. With every exhalation, let your body relax more into the pose.

Did you feel the breath doing all the work?

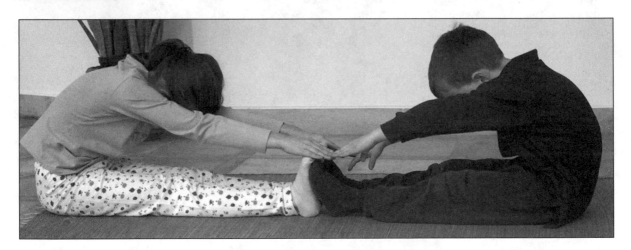

"Yes, when I concentrated on my breath, it was easy to relax more into the pose."
"The breath was my secret motor."

Snuggle Pose

BENEFITS: This pose opens the hips, tones the spine and stretches the back muscles. It also balances the energy and is emotionally nourishing.

Sit facing one another. Partner One, bend forward and turn to rest your head on your partner's knee. Partner Two, bend forward and gently rest your head on your partner's back.

Rest here breathing together for several deep breaths. With every exhalation, let yourself relax more. Think of all the people you love and concentrate on cherishing them for a few minutes.

When you are ready, come back up and reverse positions, with the other partner resting on your knee.

What did you feel?

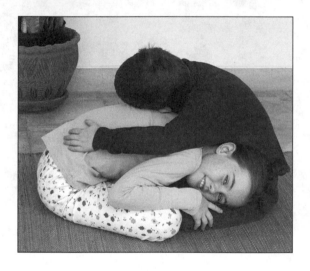
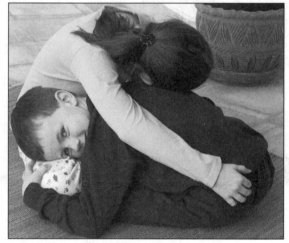

"I felt like I was giving and receiving love at the same time."

"I feel like a little lion cub being cherished by its mother."

Forward Backbend

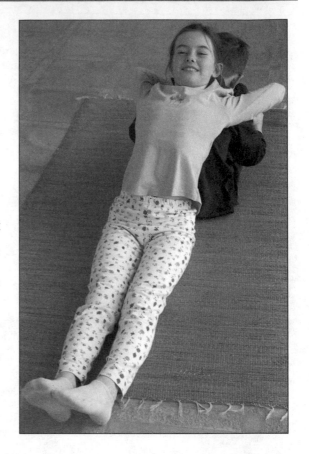

Sit back to back with your partner with your legs stretched out in front of you.

Partner One, stretch your arms up, bend your elbows and give your partner your hands. Partner Two, hold your partner's hands and slowly bend forward, allowing your partner to rest her torso and head on your back. Gently, pull your partner forward a little more with each exhalation.

Rest here, breathing together for several breaths. With each inhalation, feel the breath expand all the way down through your legs, and stretch out through the heels of your feet. Feel your chest expand and breathe into your lower back, feeling it expand against your partner's lower back. With every exhalation, let your body soften as your partner pulls you a bit further into the pose. When you are ready, slowly expand back up to center and reverse roles.

"How does it feel?"

"It feels like he's doing all the work."

"It's easy. When will we get to the hard stuff?"

Sleeping Thunderbolt

BENEFITS: The partner below is resting in the Child's Pose which stills the mind and nourishes the nerves in the muscles of the thighs. The partner on top enjoys an opening of the chest. Since his head is slightly lower than his torso, he experiences a calming, soothing effect. The reversed blood flow nourishes the brain and calms the mind. This supported pose also has a nourishing emotional effect and enhances trust between partners.

Partner One, rest in the Child's Pose, with your forehead on the floor and your arms stretched forward. Partner Two, gently sit down on your partner's lower back. Very slowly, roll back to rest your spine on hers and stretch your arms up to rest on top of your partner's hands.

Rest here, breathing together. As you breathe in deeply, visualize the breath expanding all the way through your body, into your legs and down into your feet. Feel the soles of your feet on the floor and imagine you have roots that go deep into the earth.

With each inhalation, feel your back expand against your partner's back. With each exhalation, let your body relax more.

When you are ready to come out of the pose, Partner Two, slowly roll back up to sit on your partner's lower back. Then, very gently slide off to sit on the floor.

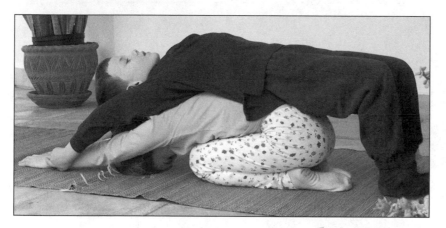

"How do you feel?"

"My body feels very relaxed."

"My mind feels very calm and happy."

Cat Stretch

BENEFITS: For the partner on top, this pose creates a wonderful opening in the abdominal muscles, shoulders, and chest. As the partner below pushes on his hands to arch his back, he uses the weight of the top partner to strengthen his arms and expand his shoulder joints. The rocking motion creates a soothing effect for both body and mind.

Partner One, come up to rest on all fours. Partner Two, gently sit down on your partner's lower back. Slowly, roll down to lie back to back with your spine in line with your partner's. Breathe in deeply. As you exhale, let your body relax completely and stretch your arms up alongside your ears.

Partner One, push your hands to arch your back like a stretching cat, allowing you to stretch your arms more. As you inhale, breathe into your lower back. Feel your back expand against your partner's back. As you exhale slowly with your partner, relax your back and stretch your tailbone toward the sky.

When you are ready to come out of the pose, Partner One, sit back in the Child's Pose so your partner may slowly roll off. If you like, reverse positions and repeat this pose.

What do you feel?

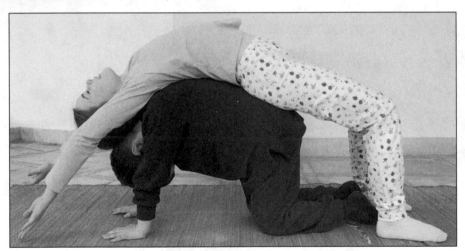

"It feels stimulating and relaxing at the same time."
"I feel the muscles in my arms getting stronger."

The Wheel

Partner One, come up to rest on all fours. Partner Two, walk to the side and gently sit down sideways on the middle of your partner's back.

Partner Two, place your feet firmly on the floor about eighteen inches apart. Slowly, rest your back across your partner's back, then raise your arms and let your head slowly stretch back. If it is easy for you, stretch your arms back and down until your hands touch the floor. Now, place the palms of your hands on the floor with your fingertips facing your feet. If your hands do not easily reach the floor, you may rest your back on your partner's back and let your arms hang to the sides.

Breathe in deeply and press on your hands and feet as you arch your trunk up as far as comfortable. Rest here, breathing deeply for a few breaths, keeping the buttocks firm and rolling the thighs in and up toward the hips. With every exhalation, open the chest more, lifting the upper arms and creating space in the shoulder joints.

When you are ready to come down, keep your arms strong as you slowly release the arch in your spine until your back again rests on your partner's back. If your spine is very flexible you may lift yourself up to sit on your partner's back and then stand up. If it is not easy for you to sit up by yourself, your partner may come down to rest in the Child's Pose with his forehead on the mat, so you may roll off.

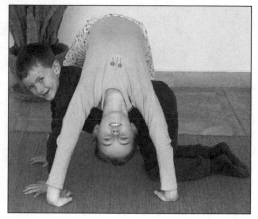

If you like, you may now reverse positions and repeat this pose.

What do you feel?

"I feel energy rising up my legs and going all the way up into my hands."
"I'm ready to be the wheel."

Andrew's Airplane

BENEFITS: Improvising allows children to develop their innate creativity, develops their ability to work together and enhances joy.

It's time to take a break from the traditional Yoga poses to improvise. It's fun to create your own poses. Like the ancient sages who created all the classic Yoga poses, you intuitively know what positions your body needs.

So, feel free to take an improvising break and create your own poses.

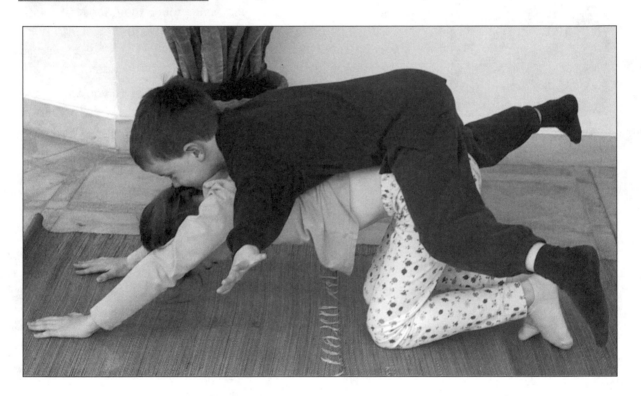

"What is improvisation?"
"Creating fast."
"Fast and fun creation!"

Andrew's Airplane

"How does it feel?"

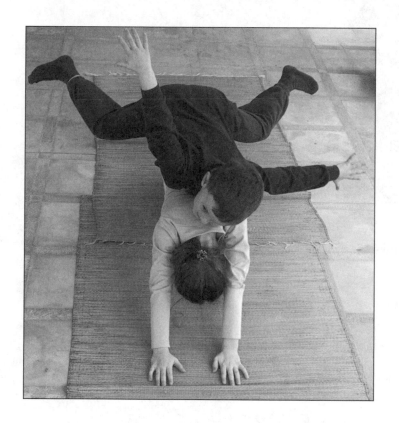

"It feels fun"

"I knew you'd like climbing on people."

Upward • Downward Dog

Partner One is resting in the Downward Dog pose, a traditional Yoga pose that calms the heart and rejuvenates the body. It stretches the spine and back muscles and relieves compression between the vertebrae. For the partner resting on top, this supported pose is restful and rejuvenating.

Partner One, rest on all fours. Then, tuck your toes under and slowly lift your hips up to rest in the Downward Dog Pose. Partner Two, stand in front of your partner and place your feet alongside her hands. Gently, sit back to rest your hips on her upper spine. Now, lie back against her back with your spine in line with hers. Inhaling, stretch your arms up alongside your ears and then reach back to place your hands on the back of her thighs.

Exhaling, let your back relax against her back and the back of your head rest on the base of her spine. As you breathe in deep, feel your shoulders expand against her lower back. As you breathe out long, stretch down through your feet and up through your head and feel your spine elongate.

Rest here for a few breaths. When you are ready, slowly stand up and reverse positions.

"What did you feel?"

"I felt like I was supporting him."
"When I trusted her, I could feel my muscles relax more."

Bowsprit Lunge

BENEFITS: This pose limbers and strengthens the entire skeletal structure. It also develops balance and concentration.

Kneel with your back facing your partner's back. Inhaling, step forward with your left foot, keeping your left knee directly over your left ankle. Exhaling, bend forward, placing your hands by the sides of your left foot.

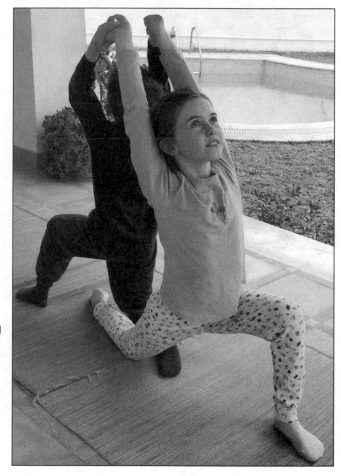

Inhaling, stretch the right leg back, keeping your arms alongside the ears as they stretch up. Exhaling, stretch your arms toward the back to take hold of your partner's hands.

Lift your chin slightly and rest here breathing together for three deep breaths. On the third exhalation release your partner's hands and slowly bend forward. Keep the arms alongside your ears and elongate your spine as you bring your hands back down by your foot.

Now, bring your left knee back beside your right one and repeat this pose with your right foot on the floor.

Imagine you standing on the bowsprit of a huge boat.

What do you feel?

"When I close my eyes, I can feel the water spray and cool wind in my face."
"I feel like I'm King of the World."

Hand To Foot Pose

BENEFITS: This pose stretches the back muscles and keeps the spine supple. The forward bending gives a massage to the abdominal organs, improving digestion and enhancing the appetite.

Stand side by side with your partner with your right foot about twelve inches away from his left foot. Separate your own feet about twelve inches apart and step your outside foot forward a bit.

Inhaling, raise your arms to the sides. Exhaling, bend forward until your outside arm touches your outside foot. Inhaling, stretch your inside arm up toward the sky and take hold of your partner's hand. Now turn your head to look at your partner. Rest here for a few breaths, gazing into your partner's eyes.

What do you see?

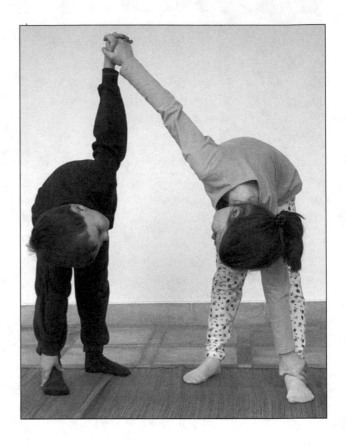

"I see the light in her eyes."
"It's like looking into a window and seeing deeper inside."

The Silent Tree

BENEFITS: The Tree Pose develops balance and concentration. It also strengthens the muscles in the legs and opens the hip joints. The ancient Yoga scriptures talk about our kinship with trees. Most children enjoy the Tree Pose, as their feeling of connection with trees is very natural.

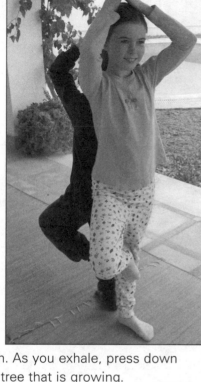

Stand back-to-back with your partner and raise one foot, placing the sole of your foot against the inside of your opposite thigh.

Inhaling, raise your arms up over your head and bring the palms of your hands together. Exhaling, press the palms of your hands together and expand up through your spine. Inhaling, breathe into the hip joint of your bent leg. As you exhale slowly, let your bent knee open back more toward your partner's bent knee.

Inhaling, breathe all the way down through the body. Imagine that your legs are the trunk of the tree, your arms the branches and your fingers the smaller twigs. Imagine that all the hairs on your head are the leaves of the tree. Listen to your leaves that are shimmering in the wind.

Now, feel the breath expand down through your trunk and into your feet. Imagine that you have roots that go deep into the earth. As you exhale, press down with your foot and feel your spine growing longer as if you are a tree that is growing.

Rest here breathing with your silent tree partner. When you feel tired, you may gently lower your arms and bring your foot down. Then, repeat the Tree Pose with the other leg.

"What is something that all trees share?"
"Their silence."
"What is the fruit of the silent tree?"
"Peace."

Tangle Foot Pose

BENEFITS: This pose stretches and strengthens the legs, opens the hips and develops balance and concentration.

Begin by standing side by side. Now step apart until your palm can rest on your partner's shoulder.

Partner One, raise your inside leg in front, allowing Partner Two to hold your foot with her outside hand. Partner Two, raise your inside leg behind Partner One, allowing him to hold your foot with his outside hand.

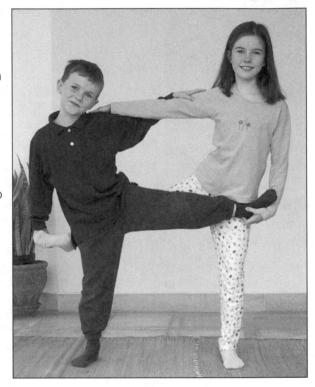

Rest here breathing together. With each inhalation, feel the breath expand down through the legs and stretch out through your extended legs. With each exhalation, try to stretch your inside hips down, until they are level with your outside hips.

On the next inhalation, let the breath expand all the way down through the standing leg and into the foot. Imagine that you have roots that go deep into the earth. On the exhalation, press your foot gently into the floor more and feel your spine expand up.

When you are ready to come down, slowly release your legs. Now, change sides and repeat this pose with your other leg.

Do you feel your roots going deep into the earth?

"I feel like even our roots are tangled together."
"When I concentrate on feeling my roots, it's easier to keep my balance."

Wheelbarrow

Partner One, lie on your stomach with your legs straight. Place your palms face down on the mat alongside your shoulders. Inhale and raise the chest and head so the back is arched. Rest here breathing deeply.

Partner Two, stand behind your partner and gently lift her feet.

Now, Partner One, balance on both arms and slowly walk forward on your hands. Partner Two, walk with her keeping her feet lifted.

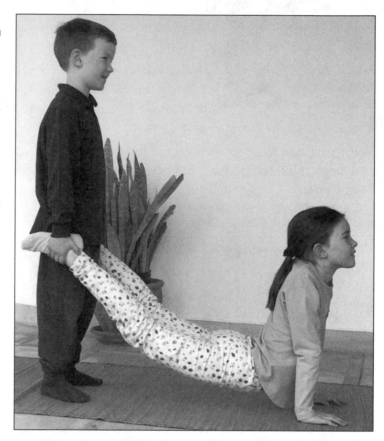

When you like, slowly lower your partner's legs, then relax and change positions.

What do you feel?

"It feels like we are a four legged animal."

"I feel my arms doing all the work."

33

Twin Turtles

BENEFITS: Practicing this pose with a partner allows the person on the bottom to take a deeper stretch and is emotionally nurturing for both partners. The Child's Pose is a great counter-pose to practice after bending backward.

Partner One, sit on your knees with your forehead on the mat and your arms alongside your body. Rest here in the Child's Pose. Partner Two, carefully climb on Partner One's back. With your knees resting softly on her back, place your hands on her shoulders and slowly bend forward to rest your forehead on her upper back.

Close your eyes and rest here for several breaths. As you breathe with your partner, relax your shoulders and neck completely.

Breathe in deeply and then concentrate on the space before the inhalation. Exhale long and then observe the space before the exhalation. Continue like this for a few deep breaths, sinking deeper and deeper into the subtle space between each breath.

When you are ready to come out of the pose, Partner Two gently slides his feet down to touch the floor and then carefully rolls off. Do you feel the space between each breath growing longer and longer?

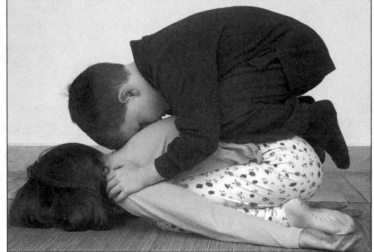

"When I concentrate completely, the space between each breath expands."

"When I go deep inside my breath, I feel the space before the inhalation connecting with the space before the exhalation."

Sleeping Stars

Lie on your back with the top of your head touching the top of your partner's head. Inhaling, stretch your arms up to hold your partner's hands. Exhaling, bend your knees and open them wide apart as you fold your legs, so your feet rest alongside your hips

With each inhalation, imagine you are expanding up into the stars. With each exhalation, sink deeper inside yourself.

Rest here, enjoying the silence that unites you and your partner. Let your awareness expand until you share this silence with all the stars.

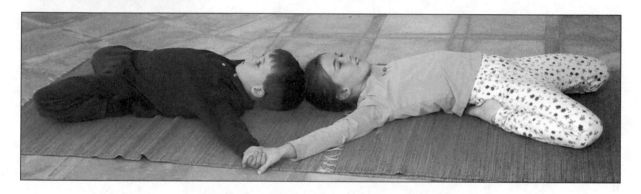

"Do you feel that we're sharing all the stars with each other?"

"It feels so soothing."

"It feels like this deep silence unites us all."

Contemplation

Visualize a beautiful pink cloud.

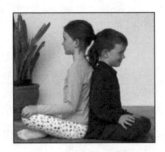

Now put your thoughts on the cloud

and let them float away.

Chapter Three

Keep Mom Young With Yoga

Play with your children rather than watch them play

"Grace, beauty, strength and energy adorn the body through Yoga."
— Yoga Sutra 111,47

Tension drains vitality. Learn to release tension and give and receive nourishment. Experience that true beauty and love emanate from within. This series of Nourishing Partner Poses is designed to inspire mothers and children to go beyond daily roles and connect on a deeper level. These playful poses will stimulate and rejuvenate every part of your body, refresh your mind and inspire your spirit.

The Rowboat

Mom sits with her legs open wide, with the soles of her feet touching her partner's soles. You and your partner sit in front of your moms with your legs open wide and the soles of your feet touching.

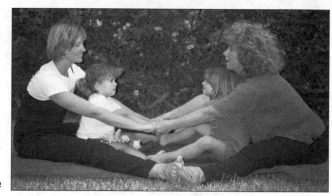

Mom holds her partner's hands and you hold your partner's hands. Inhaling, you and Mom stretch toward the back, pulling your partners forward. As you exhale your partners stretch back, pulling you and Mom forward. Continue like this, moving back and forth with each breath. Feel your spine expand as you move in one continuous motion with the breath.

Imagine you are rowing a boat across a calm blue lake. Do you feel your body rowing with each breath?

"...Merrily, merrily, merrily, life is but a dream."
"I feel our little boat gliding over the smooth lake."

Sailors' Stretch

BENEFITS: The Sailboat Stretch opens the shoulder joints, stretches the muscles in the arms and expands the spine. The twist tones the abdominal organs.

Mom sits with her legs open wide, with the soles of her feet touching her partner's soles. She twists toward the right and holds her partner's opposite hand. Inhaling, she stretches her arm toward the back as she pulls against her partner's hand. You and your friend stand behind your moms and pull their arms, helping them stretch more. Mothers rest here breathing together as you continue to pull on their hands, stretching them further.

Now, release your mom's hands for a minute, when they come back to center, she takes her partner's other hand and twists toward the left.

Again, take your mom's hand and pull toward the back. Inhaling, Mom stretches her arm back and pulls against her partner's hand. As they rest here, you continue to pull gently while your moms twist more. When they are ready to release the pose, gently let go of her hand.

Did you feel her body expand?

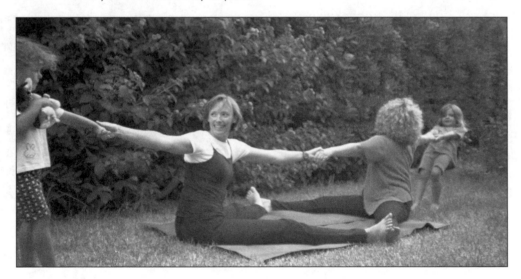

"It felt like blowing up a balloon."
"Mom's arms grew longer and longer."

The Raven

BENEFITS: This pose expands the chest and lungs, enhancing breathing capacity. It also gives a good massage to the back and stretches the spine.

Mom sits behind you with her legs stretched out in front of her. You sit in front of her feet with your legs stretched to the front. Mom places her right foot on your lower back and her left foot on the middle of your back at heart level.

As you stretch your arms toward the back and look up at the sky, Mom takes hold of your hands. As she slowly pulls your arms toward the back, imagine you are a huge raven opening your wings. As you fly up into the vast blue sky, breathe deeply into your chest.

Rest here, breathing deeply while Mom continues to gently open your wings. Let your chest expand more with each breath.

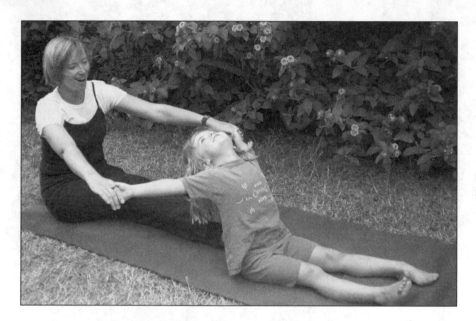

"What do you feel?"
"I feel like a beautiful bird soaring through the big blue sky."

Take me to the Sun

BENEFITS: This pose is rejuvenating for Mom, as it reverses the blood flow in her legs, relieving varicose veins. The weight of the child on her legs helps to release her hip joints and stretches the muscles in her legs, strengthening her lower back and abdomen. It also stretches and strengthens the muscles in Mom's arms and legs. Like all the supported poses, this pose is emotionally nurturing for the child. It enhances a feeling of trust and interdependence and gives the child a feeling of joy and freedom.

Mom lies down on her back and bends her knees. Gently, she puts her feet on your abdomen and holds your hands. As Mom slowly lifts you up, imagine you are flying toward the sun.

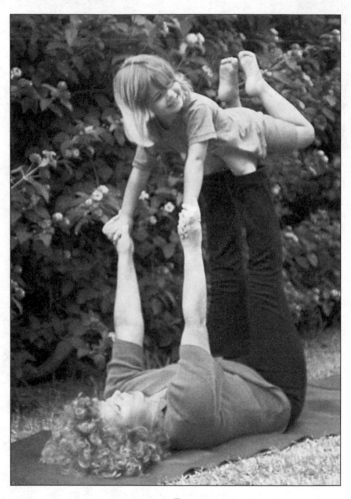

"How do you feel?"
"I feel happy and free."

The Starfish

BENEFITS: This deep forward bend is rejuvenating and restful for Mom. It stretches her legs and spine, soothes her nervous system and draws her mind inward. It is emotionally nourishing for the child who enjoys an effortless expansion of the chest and diaphragm. The reversed blood flow to the child's head also creates a soothing, calming effect.

Mom sits with her legs open and her knees bent a bit. Then she bends forward and slides her arms under her knees and holds her ankles with her hands.

You stand behind Mom and gently sit down on her back. Slowly, lie back on Mom's back with your spine in line with hers. As you breathe in deeply, feel your chest expand and let your arms relax to the sides and your head rest on Mom's head.

As you breathe out long, imagine you are a beautiful starfish swimming in the deep blue sea. As you breathe in, feel the warm ocean water washing through all your pores.

When you are ready to come out of the pose, Mom slowly comes back to a seated position, and you slide down to sit on the floor behind her.

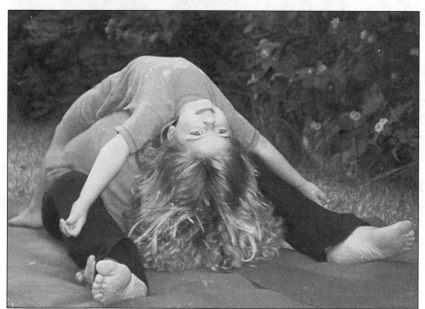

"How do you feel?"
"I feel like I'm part of the big blue sea."

The Flying Wheel

BENEFITS: The Wheel limbers and strengthens the entire skeletal structure. It opens the chest, stretches the abdominal muscles and makes the spine flexible. It develops balance and concentration and is also beneficial for the nervous and glandular systems. Like all backbends, it gives energy. Mom enjoys a rest to her legs. This pose stretches the muscles in the back of her legs, strengthens her abdominal muscles and is therapeutic for her lower back.

This pose is more advanced, so let Dad or another grown-up stand nearby to catch you if necessary.

Mom lies down on her back and bends her knees. You stand with your back facing Mom's feet and reach your arms back, so Mom may hold your hands. Gently, she places her feet on your lower back and holds your hands.

Slowly, Mom lifts you up and you arch your back until your body is like a wheel. Rest here, breathing in deep. Feel the breath expand all the way through your body, down your legs and into your feet. As you exhale, let your body relax completely.

When you are ready to come down, Mom very slowly bends her knees and brings her legs down until your feet touch the floor.

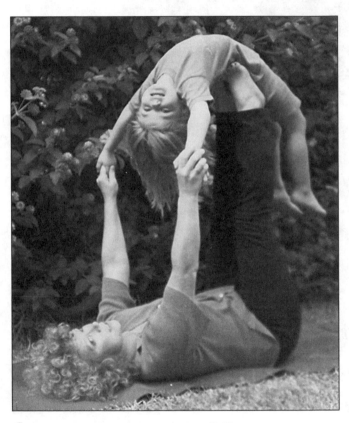

"Do you feel more expanded?"
"I feel like I'm as big as Mom."

Puppy-Back

Mom rests on all fours. You climb on her back and lie down. Wrap your arms around Mom and hold on as she tucks her toes under and slowly lifts her hips up to rest in the Downward Dog Pose.

Now you may stretch your legs out, release your arms to the sides and relax completely. As you inhale, feel your abdomen expand against Mom's back. As you exhale, let your arms and legs and torso relax even more. Imagine you are a little puppy riding on your Mom's back.

When you are ready to release the pose, Mom bends her knees to rest them on the floor in the Child's Pose. Slowly and carefully, you place your feet on the floor and stand up.

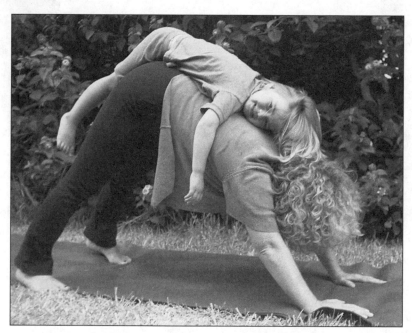

"How do you feel?"
"I feel happy and loved."

Chinese Dragon

Mom helps lift you as you jump up and wrap your legs around her waist. She holds your hips as you slowly lean backwards, hanging upside down. Place the palms of your hands on the mat with your fingertips facing Mom's toes. Now take a deep breath and push gently on your hands and feel your shoulder joints expand.

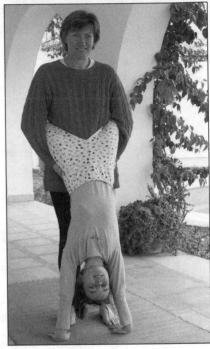

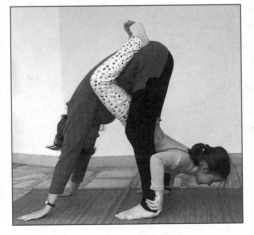

Exhale slowly, letting your body relax more into the pose. Now, reach back and grab Mom's ankles. Mom bends forward, putting her hands on the floor. As you rest here for a few breaths, imagine you are a friendly dragon.

"Can you roar playfully?"
"RRRRRR...oooo...aaaa...rrrrrrrrrrr!"

Crescent Moon

BENEFITS: Mom is resting in the Downward Dog Pose, which reverses the blood flow and brings energy to the upper body. Since it is a weight-bearing exercise for the entire body, it is an ideal pose to practice for preventing osteoporosis. The increased blood flow to the head nourishes the brain and calms the mind. It also stretches the spine and back muscles and relieves compression between the vertebrae. For the child, this stretch produces a unique release in the shoulder girdle. The polarity created when she pulls against Mom expands her spine and opens her shoulder joints. It also expands her diaphragm and chest, facilitating deeper breathing.

Mom rests on all fours. Then, she tucks her toes under and slowly lifts her hips up to rest in the Downward Dog Pose.

You stand in front of Mom and place your feet between her hands. Gently, sit back to rest your hips on her upper spine. Now, lie back against her back with your spine in line with hers. Inhaling, stretch your arms up alongside your ears and then reach back to place your hands on the back of Mom's thighs.

As you exhale, feel your entire body soften and relax against Mom's and feel the back of your head resting on the base of her spine. As you breathe in deeply, feel your shoulders expand against Mom's lower back. As you breathe out long, stretch down through your feet and up through your head and feel your spine expanding.

What do you feel?

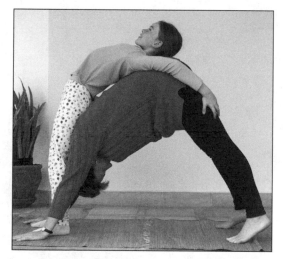

"I feel the back of my shoulders expanding against Mom's back."

"I feel energized and relaxed at the same time."

The Flowering Bridge

BENEFITS: This pose is calming, restful and rejuvenating for the child. The reversed blood flow brings and increases circulation in the brain, creating a calm, peaceful feeling. It also stretches the spine and opens the chest, creating a poised posture.

Mom rests in the Child's Pose, with her forehead on the floor and her arms stretched in front of her. You sit on her hips and stretch your torso over her back with your spine in line with hers. Breathe in deeply and stretch your arms up and hold underneath her arms with your hands. Breathe out long and let your legs stretch, feeling the tips of your toes on the floor.

Rest here for a few breaths, synchronizing your breath with Mom's breath. With each inhalation, feel your back expand against her back. With each exhalation, let your muscles soften and relax more.

With the next inhalation, breathe all the way through your body, down into your legs and into your feet. Feel the tips of your toes on the floor and imagine you have roots that go deep into the earth.

When you are ready to come out of the pose, Mom sits back on her heels so you may gently slide off to sit on the floor.

"What do you feel?"
"I feel a warm, soothing feeling."

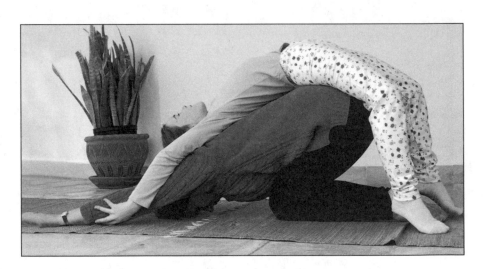

"It feels like the tension in my neck and shoulders is dissolving into the breath."

The Heavenly Pose

BENEFITS: This pose strengthens Mom's lower back and massages her spine as it allows the child to open the chest and lungs completely. The rocking motion stimulates the thousands of nerve endings in the spinal column and is calming for the child. As Mom pushes on her hands, the weight of the child strengthens her arms and opens her shoulder joints. The child enjoys a wonderful opening in the lower abdominal muscles, shoulders and chest.

Mom comes up on all fours. Gently, sit on her back placing your tailbone on top of hers. Slowly, roll back to lie down on Mom's back with your spine in line with hers. As you exhale slowly, let your body relax and your arms rest to the sides.

Now, Mom pushes on her hands to round her back allowing you to expand your chest and relax your arms more. As you inhale, breathe into your lower back. Feel your back expand against Mom's back.

Then, Mom rocks back and forth. Inhaling, she rocks back. Exhaling, she rocks forward. As Mom continues to rock back and forth, feel how this soothing rocking motion allows you to relax more.

When you are ready, Mom sits back in the Child's Pose so you may slowly roll off.

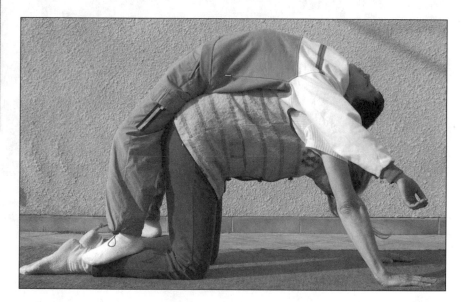

"How do you feel?"
"Like I'm having a holiday in heaven."

Kneeling Camel

Mom lies on her back and bends her knees. You kneel behind her with your back facing her feet and the tops of your feet resting alongside her hips. As she places her feet on your upper back, stretch your arms back to hold her hands.

Gently, Mom presses her feet into your back and pulls your arms toward her. Breathe in deeply and imagine you are riding through the desert on a huge camel.

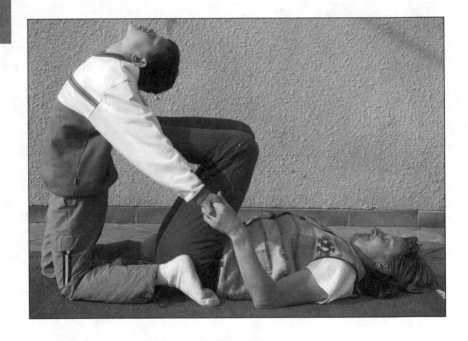

"Do you feel the silence that surrounds you?"

"Yes. Even the tiny grains of sand share the silence."

"How does it feel?"
"Soothing and peaceful."

The Flying Fish

BENEFITS: The forward bend is restful and rejuvenating for Mom, inducing a calm, meditative state. It stretches her spine and massages her internal organs. The child enjoys an effortless expansion of the chest, which enhances breathing capacity, improves posture and opens the shoulders. It gives the experience of being supported and develops trust.

Mom sits with her legs stretched to the front. You kneel behind her with your toes touching her. Mom bends forward, bringing her head toward her knees. If it is comfortable for her, she holds her feet with her hands. You lean back and lie on her back. Let the back of your head relax against her back and open your arms to the sides.

Rest here, breathing in deeply and breathing out long. On the inhalation, feel your chest expand with breath. On the inhalation, let your arms release more. Rest here as long as you like, breathing together.

What do you feel?

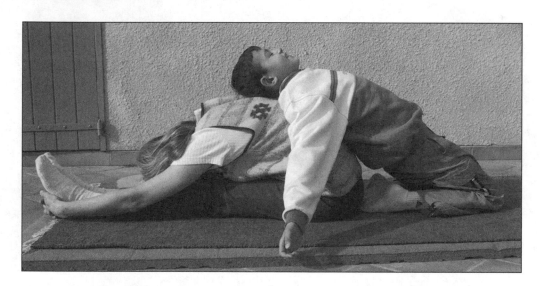

"The weight of his body makes it easier for me to go deeper into the forward bend."

"I feel my chest expanding with breath."

The Olive Press

Lie on your back with your hips touching and your hands together. Inhaling, bend your knees up into your chest and bring the soles of your feet up to press against Mom's. Rest here breathing together as you continue to gently press the soles of your feet against each other.

As you breathe in, feel the breath expand all the way through your body down into your legs and into your feet. Hold the breath in for a moment and feel your feet gently pressing against Mom's. Exhale slowly as you continue to feel the soles of your feet pressing against one another. With each exhalation, let your breath become slower and softer.

Rest here as long as you like, enjoying a few moments of silent connection.

What do you feel?

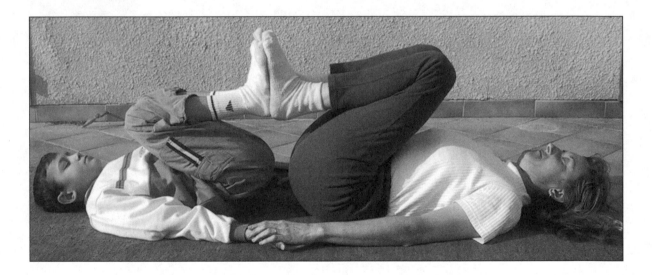

"When we inhale, it feels like Mom's breath comes in the bottom of my feet."
"I feel our love and connection."

Preparation for Spinal Column Pose

BENEFITS: This forward bend gives a massage to all the abdominal organs and stretches the muscles in the backs of the legs. It also stretches the back muscles and elongates the spine, preparing the body for the more advanced Spinal Column Pose.

Sit facing your mom with your legs stretched to the front and the soles of your feet touching. Exhaling, bend forward and take your mom's hands. If it is difficult to reach each other's hands, bend your knees a little. Rest here, with your arms alongside your ears, breathing together.

As you breathe in deep, feel the breath expand down into your legs and into your feet. Gently, press your feet against Mom's feet. As you exhale, let your body soften, allowing your abdomen to stretch toward your thighs.

Rest here a few breaths, letting the breath take you deeper into the pose. With each inhalation, feel the breath expanding your torso and spine. With every exhalation, let your body relax more.

What do you feel?

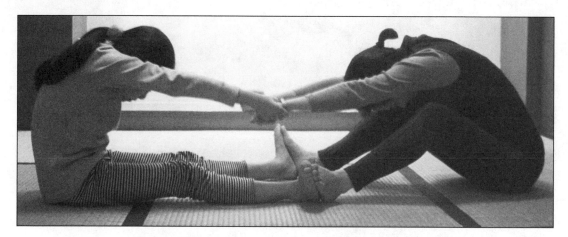

"I feel a nice stretch in the muscles in
the backs of my legs."
"I feel the tension in my neck
and shoulders dissolving."

Spinal Column Pose

Sit facing your Mom as you hold hands and bring the soles of your feet together. Gently, press your feet against your mom's feet. Slowly, raise your legs together at the same time and stretch up through the spine.

Rest here breathing together as you continue to press your feet and pull against each other's hands to keep your balance.

How do you feel?

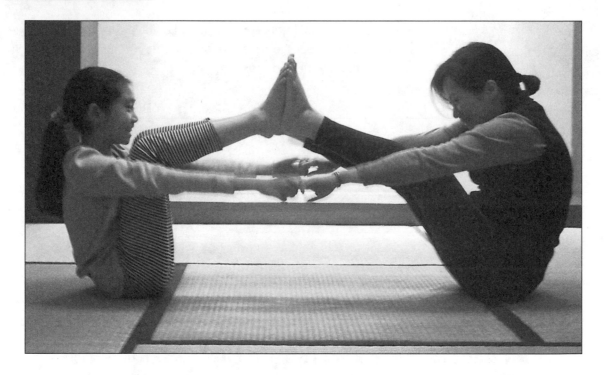

"I have to push very hard to keep my balance because Mom's legs are so strong."
"I feel like I'm young again."

Golden Door Lunge

BENEFITS: The Golden Door Lunge limbers and strengthens the entire skeletal structure. It also opens the chest, expands breathing capacity and develops balance and concentration.

Kneel with your back facing your partner's back. Inhaling, step one foot forward, keeping your knee directly over your ankle. Inhaling, stretch your arms up above your head, keeping them alongside your ears. Exhaling, stretch your arms back to hold your partner's hands.

Lift your chin slightly and rest here, breathing together. As you breathe in deeply, imagine the golden rays of the sun filling your body with its warmth and energy. As you exhale slowly, visualize

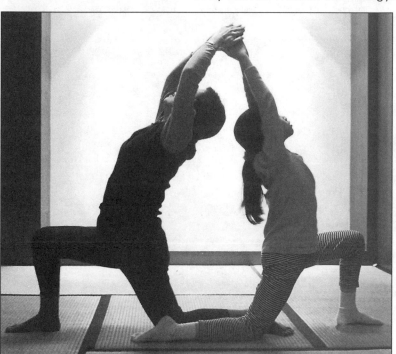

yourself radiating this warm golden energy and giving it to everyone you meet today. Rest here for several breaths, enjoying this circle of giving and receiving the golden energy of the sun.

When you are ready to change sides, slowly bend forward. Keep the arms alongside your ears and elongate your spine as you release hands and bring your arms down. Now, reverse legs and repeat this pose with your other foot on the floor.

What do you feel?

"I feel like everyday is a happy day."
"When I close my eyes, I see golden light."

The Child's Pose

BENEFITS: Mom rests in the classic Yoga pose, Child's Pose, calming both body and mind. The reversed blood flow increases circulation in the brain, creating a calm peaceful feeling. Concentrating on the space between each breath enhances our experience of the inner connection that goes beyond language.

Mom sits on her knees and brings her forehead to rest on the floor and her arms to rest alongside her body. As she rests here in the Child's Pose, you gently sit on her lower back making it easier for her to stretch her tailbone toward her feet.

As you rest here breathing together, begin to observe the space between each breath. Breathe in deeply and concentrate on the space before the exhalation. Breathe out long and concentrate on the space before the inhalation.

Rest here a few more breaths, continuing to sink deeper and deeper into the subtle space between each breath.

Now, concentrate on the silence that you share with your mom. As you sink deeper and deeper into the silent space between each breath, listen to your mom speaking without words.

Continue to rest here as long as you like, enjoying the moment of stillness between each breath.

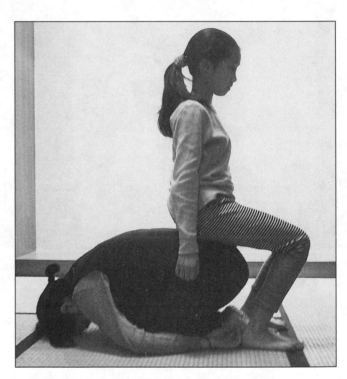

"Do you hear her silent language?"
"Yes, when I listen without ears."

Contemplation

Imagine sitting under a gentle waterfall.

Watch the water flow through your mind, washing away all thoughts.

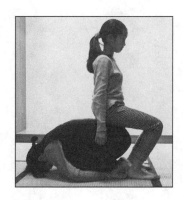

Rest here as long as you like, enjoying this state of stillness.

Chapter Four

Teach Dad to Play Yoga

You are as old as your spine

Let us walk this soft earth as relatives to all that live.

— Sioux prayer

This series of energizing partner poses are designed to keep Dad's spine young and flexible. When the spine is flexible, all the Yoga poses are easier and more beneficial because there are thousands of nerves in the spinal column that affect every part of the body. With this creative and fun approach to Yoga, your children may help you build strength and flexibility and allow you do go deeper into the poses than you could while practicing the same poses on your own. This playful partner routine will return youthful elasticity to your spine and invigorate body and mind as it gives you a new way to play with your children and bring more joy into your Yoga practice.

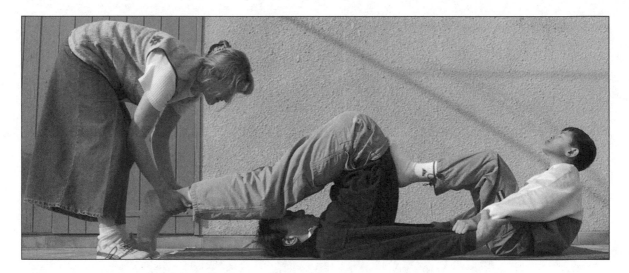

"You push and I'll pull."
"Is he getting younger yet?"

Regeneration Pose

Dad lies on his back with his hips and legs resting against your back as you sit with your legs stretched to the front. Rest here a few moments, breathing together.

On the inhalation, visualize the breath coming in the center top of your head and going all the way down the spine. Hold the breath in for a moment and concentrate on the base of the spine. Exhaling, visualize the breath expand back up through each vertebra of the spine, up through the neck and out the center top of the head. Inhaling again, observe the breath expand down the channel of the spine. Hold it in and concentrate on the tailbone. Exhaling, feel the breath expand back up through each vertebra and out the center top of the head.

Rest here as long as you like observing your breath expand up and down your spine. If you like, reverse positions and repeat this pose.

How do you feel?

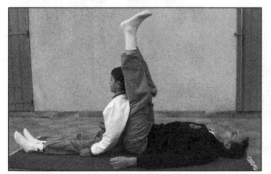

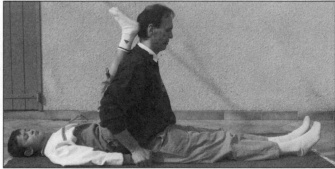

"I feel relaxed already."

"I feel like we're on the same team."

Spinal Twist

BENEFITS: The spinal twist tones the spinal nerves and massages the internal organs. It also relieves tightness in the shoulders and upper back. It has a relaxing effect on the nervous system and is beneficial for digestive ailments.

Sit facing Dad. You both bend your left legs and extend your right legs, placing the foot of your extended leg against each other's foot. As you both twist toward the right side, you hold each other's left arm.

Continue to twist as you rest here, breathing together. With each inhalation, expand up through your spine. With each exhalation, twist a little more toward the right and look to the right with your head and eyes.

Rest here as long as you are comfortable, then return to center, change legs and repeat this pose on the other side.

What do you feel?

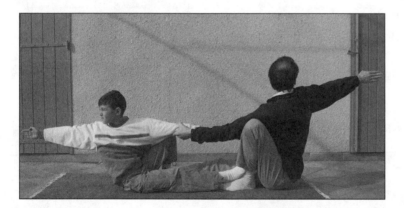

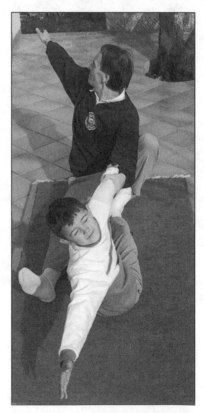

"When Dad pulls against my arm, I feel my shoulders opening."

"As we pull against each other, I feel my spine expanding."

Upside Down Bridge

Dad sits in a cross-legged position. Exhaling, he slowly bends forward as far as comfortable, bringing his arms and hands to rest on the floor in front of him. You stand in front of him, placing your feet between his hands. Gently, sit down on his shoulders. Dad holds your ankles with his hands as you slowly lie back letting your spine rest in line with his. Relax back, letting your arms open to the sides with your palms facing the sky.

Rest here, breathing together. As you breathe in deeply, feel your back expand against Dad's. As you exhale, let your muscles soften and feel your body relax more. What do you feel?

When you are ready to come out of the pose, Dad holds your ankles tightly as you slowly roll back up to sit on his shoulders and carefully stand up.

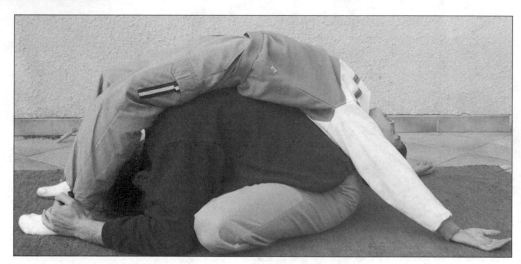

"I feel my breath opening my chest."
"His weight on my back makes it easier for me to release more forward."

Child's Pose Push-up

BENEFITS: Dad rests in the traditional Child's Pose. It stretches his spine, relieves strain in the lumbar region and gives all the muscles in the back an effortless, nourishing stretch. The weight of the child pushing allows Dad to release deeper into the pose than when he practices this pose on his own. The child strengthens his arms and upper body as he gives Dad's spine an effortless massage.

Dad rests in the Child's Pose with his forehead on the floor and his arms alongside his body. You place your hands on his upper and lower back and walk your feet back into a push-up position.

As you lift yourself up and down, doing ten push–ups, your hands press gently on Dad's spine, giving him a good massage. Come down to your knees and rest for a minute. If you like, change the position of your hands and do more push-ups until you have massaged Dad's entire spine.

How do you feel?

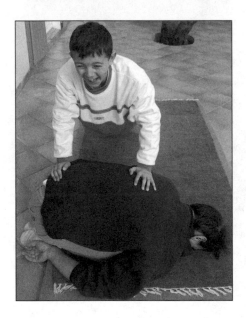 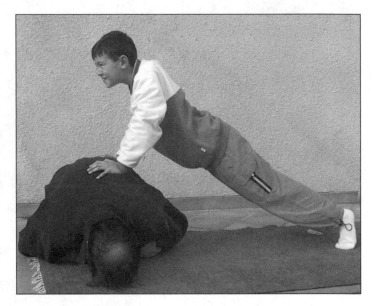

"This is fun!"
"It's a great massage!"

Dad's Wheelbarrow

BENEFITS: The wheelbarrow strengthens the muscles in the abdomen and activates the abdominal organs. It also strengthens the arms and develops balance and concentration.

Lie on your stomach with your legs bent. As you place your palms down on the mat alongside your shoulders, Dad stands behind you and lifts your feet.

Inhaling, raise your chest and head so that your back is arched. Now balance on both arms and slowly walk forward on your hands. Dad walks behind you, keeping your feet lifted.

What do you feel?

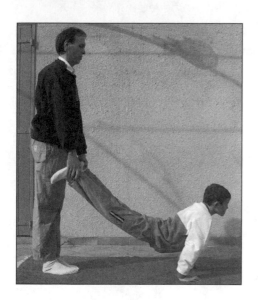

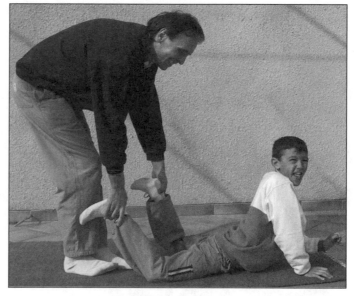

"I feel all the muscles in my arms working hard."
"My arms are working too."

Ski Lift

This pose is more advanced, so let Mom help you into the pose and stand near you to make sure you don't fall.

Dad lies on his back with his knees bent into his chest. You stand in front of Dad with your feet alongside his head. Dad lowers his feet so you may sit down on them. Mom holds you as you place your feet in Dad's hands. Dad slowly raises his feet and straightens his arms, lifting you up.

When you have your balance, Mom lets go of you but she stays close enough to catch you in case you fall. What do you feel?

To come down, Mom holds you as Dad slowly bends his knees and lowers his hands so you may place your feet on the floor alongside his head.

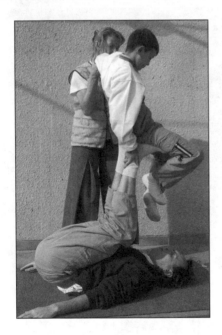

"I feel like I'm riding the ski lift up a big mountain."

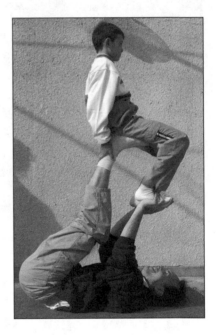

"This feels great for my lower back."

Flying Angel

BENEFITS: The Flying Angel strengthens Dad's arms, legs and lower back. It stretches the child's spine and opens the chest, creating a poised posture with an air of self-confidence and grace.

This pose is more advanced, so let Mom help you into the pose and stay nearby to catch you if necessary.

Dad stands in front of you with his knees bent. He takes your hands and helps lift you up as you place your feet on his thighs.

Inhaling, breathe through your entire body, feeling it expand.

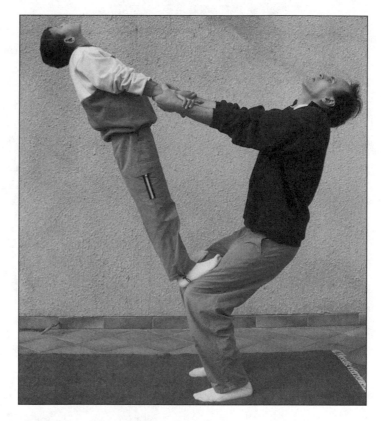

Exhaling, press your feet against Dad's thighs as you both arch your heads back as you rest here breathing together for several breaths.

When you are ready to come down, gently press your feet deeper into Dad's thighs and bring your head back up. Dad bends his knees deeper and helps you as you carefully step back down to the floor with one foot and then the other.

How do you feel?

"I feel as light as an angel."

"I feel strength rising up my spine."

Working the Plough

BENEFITS: This pose enhances the flexibility of the spine, relaxes the brain and refreshes the legs. It also strengthens the back and enhances mobility in the hip joints. It soothes and nourishes the entire body and helps the senses turn inward so the body and mind may bathe in the wellspring of joy and love within the heart.

Lie on your back and lift your legs up and over your head until the tops of your feet rest on the floor above your head. Dad sits down behind you, holds your hands and places his feet on your lower back. Rest here, breathing together.

With each inhalation, Dad gently pulls on your arms. With every exhalation, he pushes your back softly with his feet. Let yourself relax deeper into the pose with each exhalation. After several breaths, you may slowly release the pose and reverse positions. What do you feel?

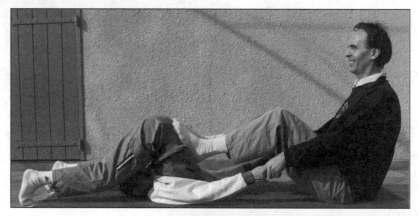

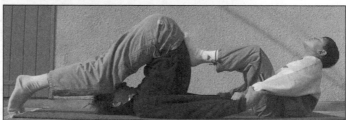

"I feel Dad's spine stretching."
"I feel much younger already."

Flying Camel

Dad lies on his back and bends his knees. You stand with your back to Dad's feet. As Dad places his feet on your upper back, stretch your arms back to hold his hands. Rest here, breathing in deeply and breathing out long together.

With each inhalation, Dad gently pulls your arms toward him. With every exhalation, he pushes softly on his feet, allowing you to arch more. Let all your muscles soften and relax as Dad pulls you gently back. Rest here, breathing deeply into your chest as long as it is comfortable. What do you feel?

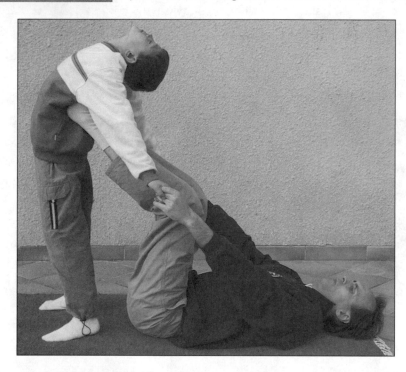

"I feel like I'm growing taller and taller."
"This feels like therapy for my lower back."

The Locust

BENEFITS: This is a partner version of the Locust, a classic Yoga pose that keeps the spine supple and tones the internal organs. It is a good counter–pose to practice after the forward bending poses. It also strengthens the back and expands the diaphragm. This version of The Locust Pose stretches the spine and strengthens the legs and lower abdominal muscles of the standing partner. It also improves posture and melts winter blues, keeping the spirit cheerful and light.

Lie on your stomach with your forehead on the floor and your arms resting alongside your body. Dad stands over you with his feet by your hips. As Dad bends his knees and places his hands on your lower back, arch up and reach your hands back to hold the back of his legs just below his knees. As Dad gently presses your hips toward the floor, lift your legs a few inches off the floor. Rest here, breathing deeply.

With each inhalation, let your entire body expand. With each exhalation, lift up a little higher. As you rest here, close your eyes and concentrate completely on your breath. When you are ready to release the pose, release your hands and roll down slowly. How do you feel?

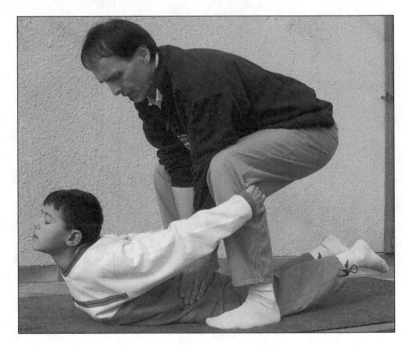

"When I pull on Dad's legs, it's easy to lift up higher."

"When I bend my knees, I feel my spine expand up."

Heavens Door

BENEFITS: Dad rests in the Child's Pose, which expands the spine, relieves strain in the lumbar region and stretches all the muscles in the back. The child enjoys an effortless opening of the torso and upper body. The reversed blood flow increases circulation in the head and brain, creating a calm, contented feeling.

Dad rests in the Child's Pose with his forehead on the floor and his arms alongside his body with his palms facing the sky. Gently, you sit down on Dad's middle back and slowly roll back to rest the top of your head on the floor. Let your arms relax to the sides with the palms of your hands facing the sky.

Rest here, breathing together. As you breathe in deeply, visualize the breath expanding all the way down the spine and concentrate on the tailbone at the base of the spine. As you exhale slowly, visualize a golden light rising up the spine like brilliant rays of the sun.

As you rest here for a few more breaths, close your eyes and imagine the warmth of the sun filling you with energy.

What do you feel?

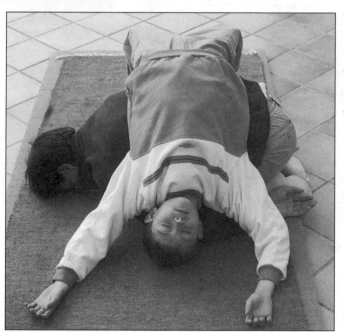

"I feel energy going down my legs, into my feet."
"It's so soothing to feel our backs breathing together."

The Huddle

Rest in the Child's Pose with the tops of your heads touching. Place your hands on each other's shoulders.

Close your eyes and rest here, breathing in deeply and breathing out long. Now begin to observe the space between each breath. Breathe in deeply, and concentrate on the space before the exhalation. Breathe out long, and concentrate on the space before the inhalation. Rest here for a few more breaths, continuing to concentrate on the subtle space between each breath.

Rest here as long as you like, enjoying the moment of stillness between each breath.

What do you feel?

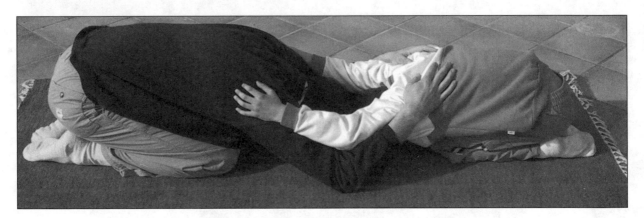

"I feel the space between each breath growing longer."

"I feel one space merging into another."

Contemplation

Imagine you are looking at a cloudless sky.

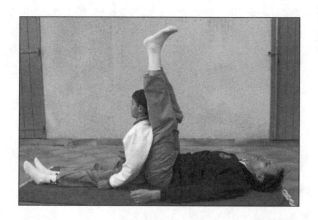

Rest here as long as you like, enjoying this stillness.

Chapter Five

Be A Fountain Of Youth For Grandma And Grandpa

Restorative Poses For The Young At Heart

"Blessed be the breath of Life who rules this world. Bring us, O Breath, your dear form, that we may live! Grant us your power to heal!"

— Arthava Veda, XI, 4

Yoga philosophy views the golden years as a time of deepening wisdom and love. As we age, the condition of our inner organs affects our state of health. This series of rejuvenating poses, designed for grandchildren to practice with their grandparents, presents a series of playful partner poses that will create healthy inner organs and a strong glandular system. This "fountain of youth" routine includes breathing techniques that enhance vitality, allowing the vital force to flow through all the organs, glands and systems of the body undiminished.

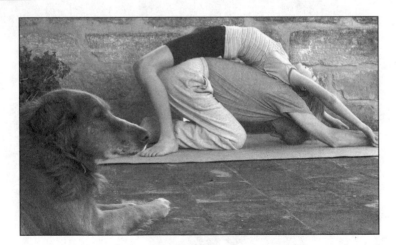

"Grandpa, Caramel looks like he's doing almost the same pose as you."
"He wants to stay young too."

Vitalizing Breath

BENEFITS: This simple breathing exercise expands breathing capacity, soothes the nervous system and revitalizes the body and mind.

Begin by sitting back-to-back, with your legs crossed. Let the palms of your hands rest gently on your knees. Take a few minutes to concentrate on your breath and synchronize your breath with your grandfather's breath. Exhale together, breathing through the nostrils. Inhaling, breathe in deeply, filling the body with breath and energy. Again, exhale long and slowly. On the next inhalation, breathe into your back and feel the breath expand your back against your grandfather's back. Continue to synchronize your breath, enjoying a few minutes of silent connection.

What do you feel?

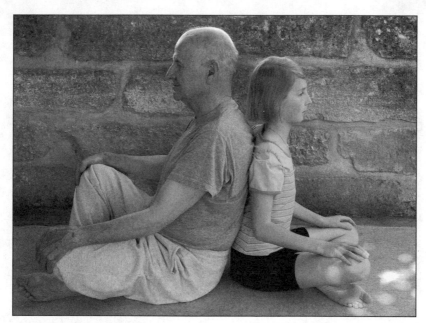

"It feels like we're sharing the same breath."
"I realize that the silent connection is always there, but often we're too busy to notice."

Arm Stretch

Inhaling, raise your arms up behind your head so Grandpa may hold your hands. Exhaling, Grandpa bends his arms at the elbows and gently stretches your arms as he slowly bends forward. With each inhalation breathe in deeply, letting your chest and shoulders expand with breath. With each exhalation feel your body soften and surrender more to the stretch.

Rest here for several breaths, allowing each exhalation to take you into a deeper stretch. When you are ready, slowly expand back to center and reverse positions.

What do you feel?

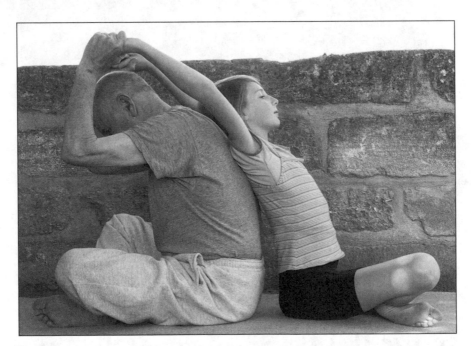

"I feel the breath expanding my ribs and chest."
"I feel our shoulders breathing together."

Long Leg Stretch

Sit back-to-back and stretch your legs toward the front. Breathe in deeply and raise your arms up behind your head so Grandpa my hold your hands. Exhale long, as Grandpa bends his arms at the elbows and slowly bends forward, giving your arms and torso a good stretch.

Rest here, breathing together. With each inhalation, let the breath expand into your chest and all the way down into your legs and feet. With each exhalation, feel your body soften and surrender to a deeper stretch.

When you are ready, Grandpa slowly expands back up to center so you may reverse roles and stretch him forward.

What do you feel?

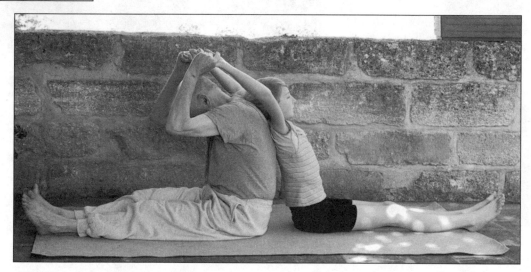

"When I breathe into my legs, it feels like they are growing longer."
"Her weight makes it easier for me to stretch deeper into the forward bend."

The Toboggan

Grandpa sits behind you and places his left foot on your lower back and his right foot on the center of your back at heart level. As you stretch your arms back toward him, he holds your hands and pulls gently.

Inhaling, breathe into your chest. As you exhale together, Grandpa softly presses his feet more into your back to enhance the stretch.

Exhaling, he gently pulls your arms back a bit more. Rest here, breathing together. With each inhalation, let you spine expand. With each exhalation he pulls gently, allowing you to relax more into the pose.

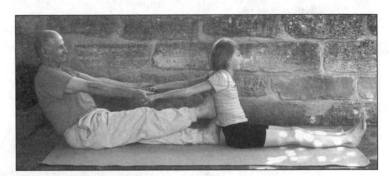

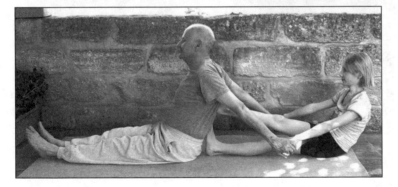

When you are ready, release your hands and turn around to reverse positions.

What do you feel?

"I feel a wonderful opening in my shoulders and chest."
"I feel Grandpa's shoulders expanding more with each exhalation."

The Bridge

BENEFITS: Grandpa rests in the Child's Pose. For the grandchild, the reversed blood flow to the head creates a calm, peaceful feeling. It also stretches the spine and expands the chest, creating a poised posture. The spinal breathing technique enhances circulation to the thousands of nerve endings in the spine, energizing the entire body.

Grandpa rests in the Child's Pose, with his forehead on the floor and his arms stretched forward. Gently, you sit down on his lower back. Slowly, roll back to rest your back on his and stretch your arms up until your fingers touch his arms.

Rest here, breathing together. As you breathe in deeply, visualize the breath expanding all the way down the spine. Hold the breath in for a moment and concentrate on the tailbone at the base of the spine. As you exhale slowly, imagine golden light rising up the spine like brilliant rays of the sun.

Rest here for a few more breaths imagining the warmth of the sun expanding through your entire body.

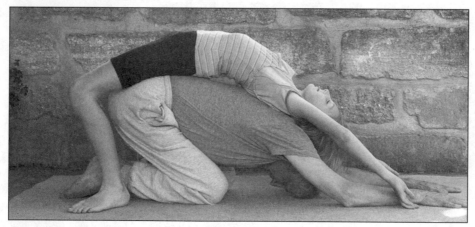

Do you feel the golden light of the sun energizing you?

"I feel it going down my legs and into my feet."
"I feel it rising up my spine."

Yin/Yang Pose

BENEFITS: This pose is restful, rejuvenating and tones the body with minimum effort. As Grandpa pushes on his hands, the weight of his grandchild strengthens his arms and opens his shoulder joints. The arching motion stimulates the thousands of nerve endings in the spine, strengthens the lower back and is soothing and relaxing. The grandchild enjoys a wonderful expansion in the lower abdominal muscles, shoulders and chest.

Grandpa rests on hands and knees. You sit on his lower back, placing your tailbone on his. Slowly lie down on his back and let your arms relax to the sides. Breathe in deep together.

Exhale slowly as Grandpa pushes on his hands to round his back. Rest here, breathing together for a few deep breaths.

When you are ready to release the pose, Grandpa sits back into Child's Pose while you slowly roll back up.

What do you feel?

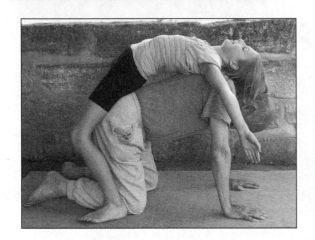

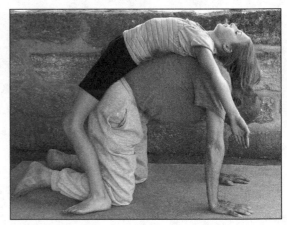

"It feels so soothing and relaxing."
"I feel my lower back expanding with breath."

Touching the Trees

Stand back-to-back. As you inhale together, Grandpa raises his arms up to rest alongside his ears and you raise your arms up and place your hands on his arms. Exhaling, Grandpa gently stretches his arms up, creating a deeper opening in your shoulder joints.

Rest here breathing together for several breaths. With each inhalation, let the breath expand all the way through the body and down into the feet. With each exhalation, stretch up more.

What do you feel?

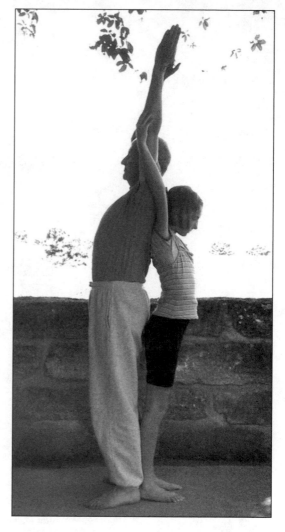

"I feel an expansion in my shoulders and chest."
"I feel the breath going all the way down to my toes."

Back-to-Back Twist

Stand back-to-back. Inhaling, raise your arms to the sides and place your hands on the inside of Grandpa's arms. Exhaling, twist to one side. Inhaling, twist to the opposite side. Continue like this for several breaths, moving from side to side in one continuous motion with the breath.

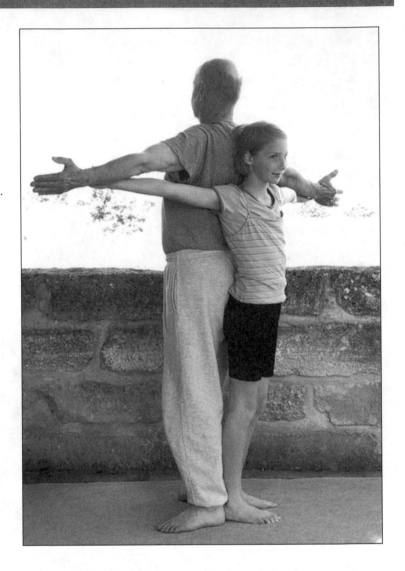

"What do you feel?"

"I feel my arms expanding."

"I feel my breath going all the way out to my fingers."

Mini Triangle

BENEFITS: This is a simple version of the Triangle Pose, a traditional Yoga pose that strengthens the legs, opens the shoulders and releases the hip joint. It also dissolves tension in the shoulders and neck, expands the spine and tones the spinal nerves. It stimulates the appetite and improves digestion. Practicing this pose with a partner makes it easier to keep the body in one plane and perform this pose with proper alignment.

Stand back-to-back with your feet about four feet apart. Open your arms to the sides at shoulder level and stretch them to the sides. Rest here a few moments synchronizing your breath.

On the inhalation, breathe in deeply, expanding your entire body with breath. Exhaling, bend down toward one foot and hold Grandpa's lower hand. Inhaling, stretch your other arms up, place your hand on Grandpa's upper arm and look up. Gently, press your back and hips against Grandpa's back and hips.

Rest here, breathing in deeply and breathing out long. Continue to stretch up through your top hand and down through your bottom hand. At the same time, elongate your spine and stretch up through your head. As you rest here breathing together, press your lower palm against your Grandfather's palm and rotate your chest toward the sky.

When you are ready, expand back up slowly and repeat this pose to the other side.

What do you feel?

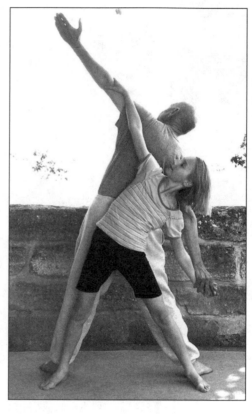

"I love feeling our backs breathe together."
"It's easier to keep my hips aligned properly than when I practice this pose myself'"

Tango Twist

BENEFITS: The Tango Twist tones the muscles of the arms, opens the shoulder joints, and strengthens the legs and lower body. It creates a lightness of spirit and is a great for melting winter blues.

Stand back-to-back with your feet about four feet apart. Inhaling, stretch your arms to your sides at shoulder level.

Exhale and clasp hands. Turn your front foot toward the front 90 degrees and your back foot facing slightly in. Inhaling, stretch your front hand behind your back, toward your back leg, as you rotate your torso to face your partner.

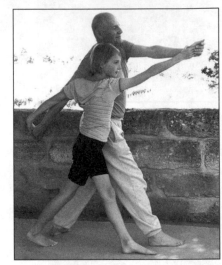

Exhaling, raise your back arm up and stretch it to the front. Rest here, breathing together. Adjust your feet so your hips are touching and extend your front arm to the front and your back arm to the back. Enjoy the stretch all the way down the inside of your arm. On the inhalation, pull your tailbone down to elongate your spine.

As you expand up through the top of your head and down through the base of your spine, stretch out from side to side with your arms. Rest here with your body still as a mountain and your breath flowing like a dancer. Breathe down into your feet and feel the muscles in your legs wrapping around the leg, bringing the energy up through your body as you stretch out from side to side with your arms.

When you are ready to come out of the pose, lower your front arm and lift your back arm up toward the sky. Exhaling, release your front arm and swing back around to stand back to back with your partner. Rest here a few moments observing your breath and the warmth in your shoulder joints. Then, repeat the Tango Twist to the other side. What do you feel?

"I feel my shoulders opening and my arms expanding from side to side."

"It feels like we're doing an inner tango."

Supported Shoulder Stand

BENEFITS: This pose, like all the inverted poses, revitalizes the entire system. It improves circulation and takes your weight off the legs. Since it reverses the blood flow and increases circulation to the brain, it helps concentration and improves our ability to sleep well. It also tones the glandular system and activates the pituitary gland. Practicing it with a partner gives physical and psychological support and makes this more advanced pose easier and safer to learn.

Grandpa lies on his back with his arms to the sides and his knees bent into his chest. You lie down in front of his feet, with your hips close to his. Now, support your hips with your hands as you lift your legs up into the shoulder stand.

Grandpa lifts his legs and places the soles of his feet on your buttocks. As he gently pushes with his feet, lift your legs up until they are as vertical as possible. As you rest here, bring your arms down to rest on the mat with your elbows bent and your palms facing the sky. Breathe deeply together for several breaths. With each inhalation, feel your breath expanding up into your feet, lifting your legs more toward the sky. With every exhalation, let your body relax more into the pose.

When you are ready to release the pose, bend your knees and slowly roll down, bringing your feet to the floor. If you like, reverse positions and repeat the pose.

What do you feel?

"His support allows me to hold this pose with an effortless feeling."

"I feel the power of a supporting relationship."

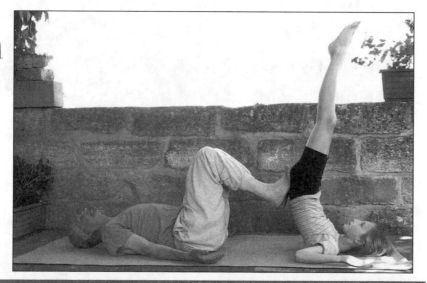

Pulling the Plow

Lie down on you back, bend your knees, support your hips with your hands and roll up to bring your knees alongside your ears into the Plough Pose. Stretch your arms behind you and out to the side so Grandpa may scoot in to sit between your arms so his back is gently pressing against your back, helping you go deeper into the stretch. As you breathe in deeply, Grandpa pulls your hands toward him, allowing you to expand your shoulder joints.

Rest here for a few breaths, feeling your backs breathe together. With each inhalation, feel the breath expanding your backs against each other. With each exhalation, feel the muscles in the back soften. When you are ready to release the pose, Grandpa moves forward, so you may roll back down.

How do you feel?

"When he pulls my arms, I feel my knees touching the floor more."

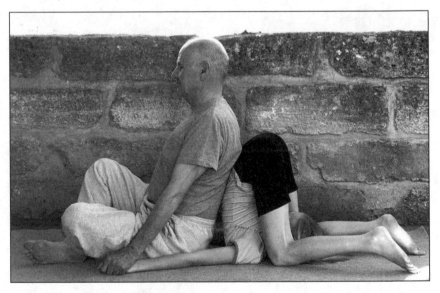

"It's more relaxing than plowing my vineyard and I feel the preciousness of this moment."

Breathing Together

Sit facing each other, with your legs crossed. Reach forward with your arms to hold each other's wrists. Inhaling, breathe in deeply, expanding the body with breath and energy. Exhale together, long and slowly. On the next inhalation, visualize the breath coming in the center top of your head and expanding all the way down the spine. Hold the breath in for a moment and concentrate on the tailbone at the base of your spine. Exhaling slowly, visualize the breath expanding up through each vertebra and out the center top of your head. Rest here for several breaths and continue to synchronize your breath with your grandmother's breath.

As your breath expands up and down the spine, do you feel an inner expansion?

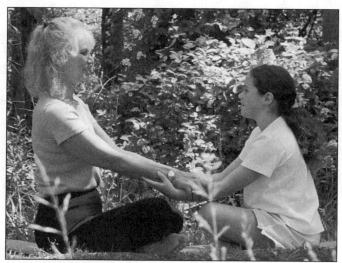

"It feels like my spine is growing."
"I feel the breath creating a space between each vertebra."

Gemini Pose

BENEFITS: This pose stretches the side of the body, slims the waist and creates a release in the hip joint. It also expands the diaphragm, enhancing breathing capacity.

Sit facing each other and stretch one leg forward bringing the sole of your foot to touch Grandma's sole. Bend your other leg at the knee and place your foot on the inside of your thigh.

Breathe in deeply as you bend forward, stretching your hand toward your feet and raising your outside arm. Rest here, breathing together for several breaths. With each inhalation, feel the breath expanding your raised arm more toward the sky. With every exhalation, feel your hip joint releasing, allowing you to stretch more toward each other's foot.

When you are ready, expand back up to center, change legs and repeat this pose to the opposite side. What do you feel?

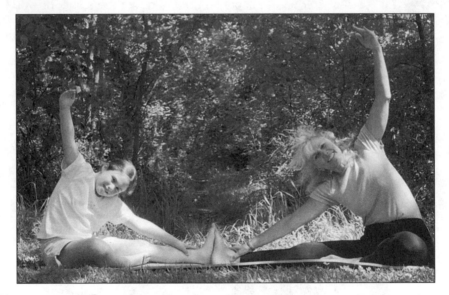

"I'm so lucky to have a Nana who is so young and healthy."

"I feel a deep stretch in my shoulders and waist."

84

Double Diamond

Sit facing each other and stretch one leg forward bringing the sole of your foot a few inches from Grandma's sole. Bend your other leg at the knee and place your foot on the inside of your thigh.

Exhaling, bend forward and try to touch the foot of your extended leg. Inhaling, stretch your other arm up and to the side and press the palm of your hand against Grandma's palm.

Rest here, breathing in deeply and breathing out long. With each inhalation, feel the breath expanding your arms from side to side. With each exhalation, let your body release more forward over your extended leg.

What do you feel?

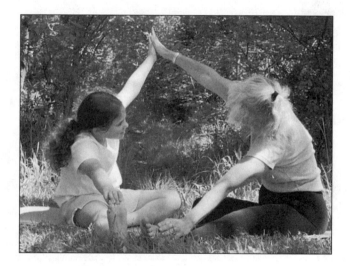

"When I stretch against Nana's palm, I feel my spine expanding."

"As we press against each other's palms, it makes it easier to bend forward."

Deep Hip Release

BENEFITS: This pose creates a deep release in the hip joints and strengthens the legs. For the grandchild, it stretches the muscles in the back of the legs and is emotionally nurturing.

Grandma lies on her back with her knees bent into her chest. You kneel in front of her and slowly place your upper body on her legs. You place your hands on Grandma's shoulders and she places her hands on your back.

As you inhale together, Grandma slowly brings her knees deeper into her chest as you stretch your legs and come up to rest on your tiptoes.

Rest here breathing together for several breaths. With each inhalation, Grandma breathes deep into her hip joints. With each exhalation, she feels her hip joints release more.

How does it feel?

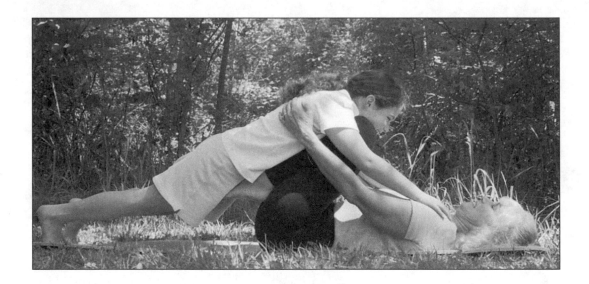

"It feels like an easy push-up."
"Her weight creates a deep, effortless release in my hip joints."

Cobbler's Stretch

BENEFITS: The Cobbler's Pose is a traditional Yoga pose that releases the hip joints. The rocking motion enhances the extension in the spine, stretches the inner thigh muscles and encourages breathing into the back of the body.

Sit facing each other in the Cobbler's Pose, with the soles of your feet together and your toes touching Grandma's toes. Stretch your arms forward to take hold of each other's wrists.

With each breath, rock forward and back. Inhaling, Grandma gently leans back, pulling you toward her. Exhaling, you lean back, pulling Grandma toward you. As you continue to move back and forth in a continuous motion with the breath, elongate your spine. Continue like this for several breaths.

What do you feel?

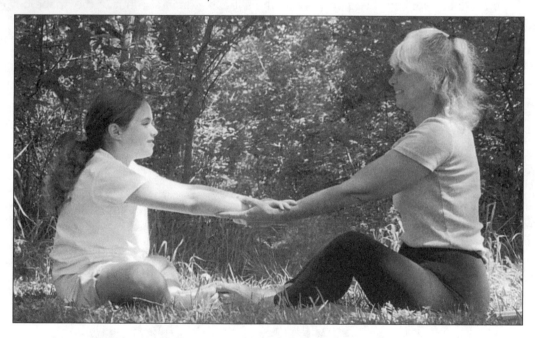

"I feel my shoulders expanding."
"I feel my hip joints releasing as we move back and forth."

Fountain of Youth

Rest on your knees and bring your foreheads on the floor, then slowly scoot toward one another until the tops of your heads touch lightly. Let your arms rest alongside your body, with the palms of your hands facing the sky.

Rest here a few moments, synchronizing your breath. Concentrate completely on the breath. On the inhalation, close your eyes and bring your awareness to the space between the eyebrows. Inhaling, imagine you are opening a window in the space between the eyebrows and breathe in there. Exhaling, observe the breath stream out the space between the eyebrows. Continue to rest here concentrating on the breath as it expands in and out of the space between the eyebrows.

With each inhalation, feel the breath come in the space between the eyebrows and expand through your entire body. With each exhalation, let the breath become slower and softer. Rest here for several breaths, concentrating on the subtle stream of breath as it comes in and out the space between the eyebrows.

How do you feel?

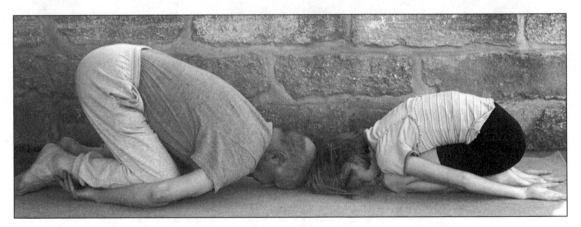

"I'm lucky to have a Grandfather who does Yoga."
"I feel like everything has dissolved into the breath."

Contemplation

Imagine being reunited with
someone you love.

Concentrate on the delight
you feel.

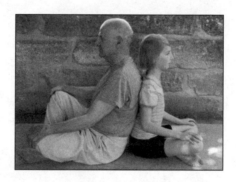

Now, let the image of your
loved one dissolve and
experience how the feeling
of delight and love comes
from within your own heart.

Chapter Six
Sweet Dreams

Prepare for a deep, restful sleep as you end the day together

Be still. Stillness reveals the secrets of eternity.
—Tao Te Ching

When day meets night, it's time for shifting gears. This evening relaxation and slow stretch routine reveals how to wind down from a busy day and prepare for a restful sleep. In this bedtime routine, we will learn to use the breath to relax the body and experience that when the breath slows down, the mind becomes calm. Through a series of soothing postures and breathing techniques, we will uncover the calm, peaceful state that is our true nature.

You may guide your children through this routine or practice it as a family. It may be especially beneficial for children and parents to do together, inspiring them to go beyond daily roles and patterns and connect on a deeper level. Parents may also enjoy doing this routine together, after the kids have gone to bed.

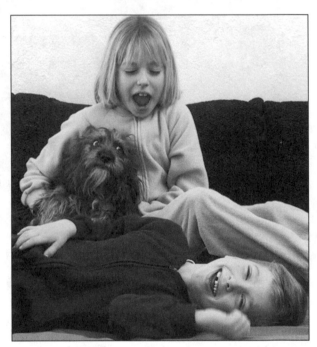

"Shall we read a bedtime story?"
"Mmmm...let's do Sweet Dreams Yoga."

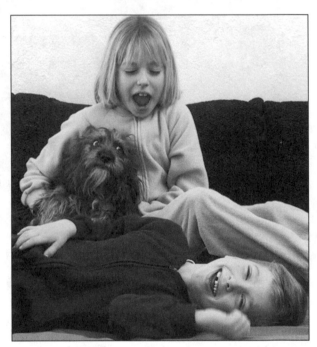

The Stick Pose

BENEFITS: The Stick Pose opens the knee joints, stretches the legs and expands the spine. It also develops the ability to breathe deeply and enhances concentration. This simple warm-up pose unites body, mind and breath which is one of the main goals of Yoga.

Sit back to back with your partner and stretch your legs out in front of you. Breathe in deeply and feel your back expand against your partner's as the back of your heads touch gently.

As you inhale, let the breath expand all the way down through your legs and into your feet. Exhaling, feel the breath expanding up your spine, making you taller. Continue to breathe like this for three deep breaths.

Imagine that your legs are sticks that grow longer with each inhalation. Feel your spine expanding with each exhalation.

What do you feel?

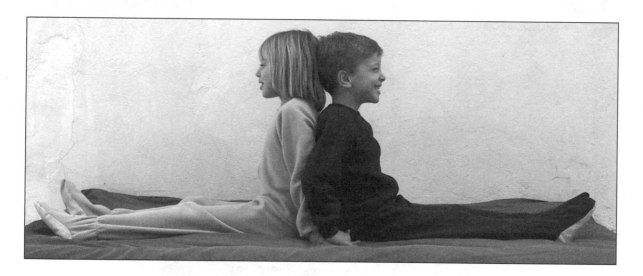

"My legs feel straight as sticks."
"I feel myself growing up through my head and
out through my feet at the same time."

Chaise Longue

BENEFITS: The Chaise Longue Pose gives a rest to the heart and drains the lymph glands in the legs. It rejuvenates the body and calms the mind. This inverted position takes the weight off the legs, tones the internal organs and prepares both body and mind for a deep, restful sleep.

Partner One, sit with your legs stretched out in front of you. Partner Two, lie down on your back with your hips touching your partner's lower back and the backs of your legs resting against his upper back and head.

Breathe deeply and feel the breath expand through your body and into your legs and feet. As you exhale, let all your muscles soften and feel yourself sinking deeper into the mat. Feel how this pose reverses the blood flow in your body, giving your heart a rest and making you feel very serene.

Rest here as long as you like, then change positions and repeat this pose.

How do you feel?

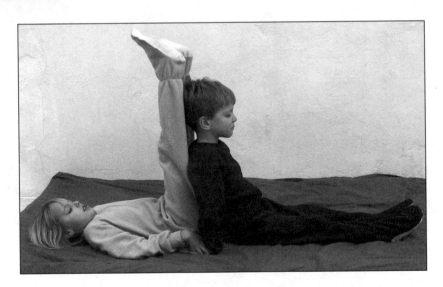

"My legs feel as light as feathers."
"Her legs make a comfortable chair for my back."

The Steeple

BENEFITS: The Steeple Pose reverses the blood flow in the body, giving a rest to the heart and calming the mind. It also stimulates the thyroid and parathyroid glands which regulate metabolism. This inverted pose takes the strain off the legs, improves circulation and tones the glandular system. It also aids concentration as blood circulation in the brain is enhanced. This pose prepares the body and mind for a restful sleep.

Lie on your back with the top of your head gently touching your partner's. Inhaling, stretch your arms to the sides to hold your partner's hands. Exhaling together, lift your hips up off the mat and raise your legs until your toes touch your partner's toes.

Rest here, breathing together. As you inhale, breathe in deeply and feel the breath expand up through your legs, lifting them up higher. As you slowly exhale, let the muscles in your shoulders and back melt into the mat. Continue to rest here as long as comfortable.

What do you feel?

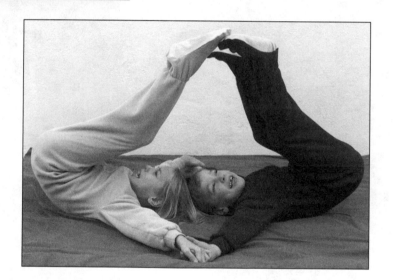

"Happy to be upside down."
"It's easier to balance when we gently press our feet against each other."

The Resting Steeple

When you are ready to come down, slowly lower your legs and then roll to the side. Rest here a few minutes imagining that you are a tired steeple that is taking a nap.

How do you feel?

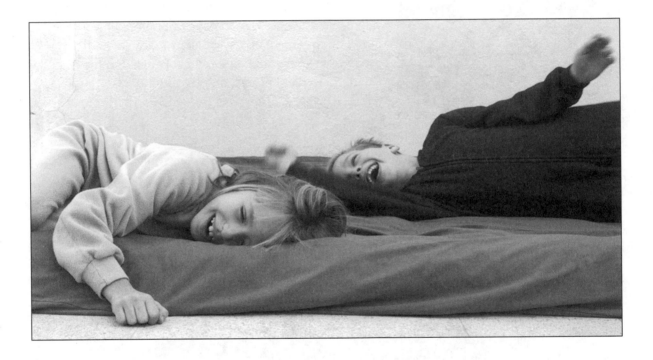

"Happy to have a long rest."

"I'm dreaming of growing into a skyscraper steeple someday."

The Bow and Arrow

Sit side by side with your partner with your legs stretched forward. Stretch your outside leg forward and stretch your inside leg toward your partner. With your outside hand, reach toward the center to hold your partner's hand.

Breathe in deeply and raise your inside hand up alongside your ear. Exhaling, stretch forward over your outside leg. Rest here for several breaths. With each inhalation, stretch up through your arm more. With each exhalation, let your muscles relax so your hand comes closer toward your foot.

Rest here as long as you like. When you are ready, you may change places and repeat this pose with your other leg.

What do you feel?

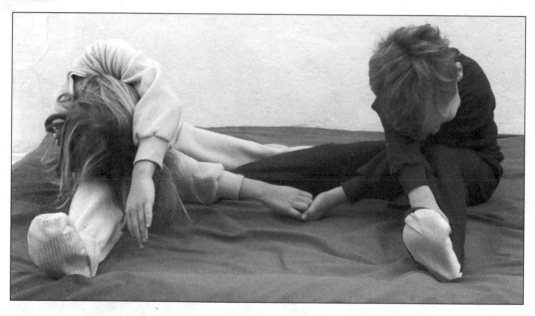

"I feel my body stretching like a bow."
"My arm feels straight as an arrow."

Laughing Cobra

Partner One, lie on your stomach with your forehead on the mat. Partner Two, stand over your partner with each foot on the outside of his knees. Bend your knees and reach your arms down to take hold of your partner's hands.

Partner One, stretch your arms back so your partner may hold your hands. Partner Two, gently pull your partner up as he lifts his head and chest up like a cobra.

Rest here for three deep breaths. With each inhalation, the cobra lifts a little higher. With each exhalation, he laughs.

When you are ready, slowly exhale as you roll back down.

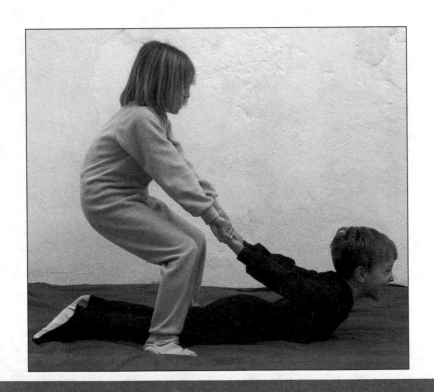

Striking Cobra

Partner Two, breathe in deeply and stretch your legs so you may pull your partner up as far as possible. Partner One, raise your chest and head as high as comfortable. Hold the breath for a moment and imagine you are a cobra ready to strike.

When you are ready to release the pose, exhale and bend your knees as you slowly lower your partner back down.

Now, change positions and let the other partner be the cobra. Will she be so friendly?

How do you feel?

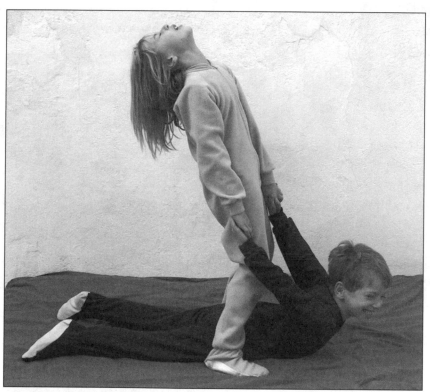

"I'm afraid he will bite me."
"I won't bite. I feel like a friendly cobra."

Sleeping Turtles

BENEFITS: This is a double version of the Child's Pose, a traditional Yoga pose that relaxes the body and calms the mind. Practicing this pose with a partner allows the person on the bottom to take a deeper stretch and is emotionally nurturing for both partners. It is a great counter-pose to practice after bending backward.

Partner One, sit on your knees with your forehead on the mat and rest here in the Child's Pose. Partner Two, carefully climb on Partner One's back. With your knees resting softly on her back, place your hands on her shoulders and slowly bend forward to rest your forehead on her upper back.

Close your eyes and rest here for several breaths. As you breathe with your partner, let yourself relax completely. Breathe in deeply, and observe the breath expand all the way down your spine. Concentrate on your tailbone for a moment. Then, as you exhale, visualize the

breath expand all the way up your spine and out the top of your head.

Breathe in deeply and then concentrate on your tailbone. Exhale long, and then observe the breath as it expands up your spine. Continue like this for a few deep breaths, sinking deeper and deeper into the breath.

What do you feel?

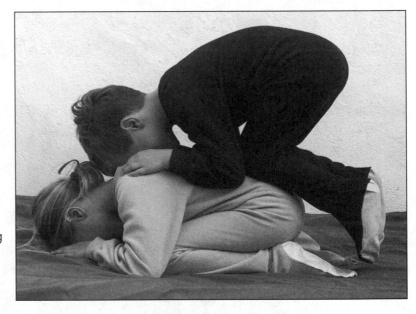

"When I concentrate on my breath, everything else disappears."
"I feel like I'm diving deeper and deeper inside my breath."

Tumbling Turtles

When you are ready to come out of the pose, you may very gently tumble off onto the mat. If you like, reverse positions and repeat the Sleeping Turtle Pose with the other partner on top.

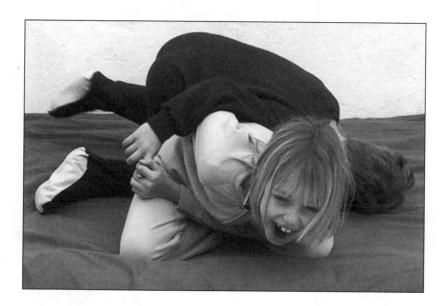

The Stork Pose

BENEFITS. This pose develops balance and concentration, strengthens the legs and enhances coordination.

Stand against the wall about three feet away from your partner. Now turn to face your partner. Stand tall with your feet together. Slowly, lean forward and raise your outside leg to the back. Try to keep your leg in a straight line with the trunk and head. Continue to bend forward until you may easily place your hands on your partner's shoulders. Now, very gently bring the tops of your heads together.

Rest here breathing together. With each inhalation, feel the breath expand all the way down into your foot. Concentrate on letting the breath expand all the way through your raised leg making it lighter. With each exhalation, feel the breath lifting your leg a little higher.

When you are ready, exhale as you slowly lower your leg. Now, change positions and repeat this pose with your other leg.

What do you feel?

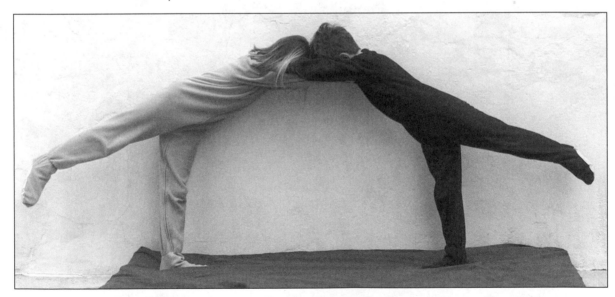

"I feel like my breath is lifting my leg."
"I feel like we're two storks telling secrets."

Double Dancers

Stand on the floor facing your partner. Lift your arm that is closest to the wall and hold hands with your partner. Keep your hand about level with the top of your head. This will help you keep your balance as you lift your opposite leg, bend the knee and hold your ankle with your hand.

As you balance here, breathe down through your leg and into your foot. Imagine that you have roots that go deep into the earth. Rest here for several deep breaths, then slowly release your arm and leg, reverse positions and try it with your other leg.

How does it feel?

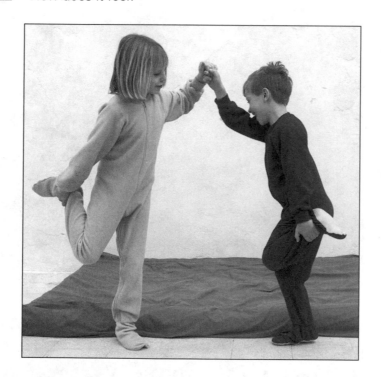

"When we concentrate we can help each other balance."
"It feels like we're silent dancing."

Wall Flowers

BENEFITS: This pose tones the muscles of the hips, legs, and feet. It also improves posture and keeps the spirit cheerful and light.

If you found it tricky to balance in the Double Dancer's Pose, stand with your foot and leg as close to the wall as possible. Lift your arm that is closest to the wall and hold hands with your partner. Keep your hand about level with the top of your head and let the outside part of your arm and leg rest against the wall. This will help you keep your balance as you lift your opposite leg, bend the knee and hold your ankle with your hand.

As you balance here, breathe down through your leg and into your foot. Imagine that you have roots that go deep into the earth. Rest here as long as you like, then slowly release your arm and leg. Then reverse positions and try it with your other leg.

How do you feel?

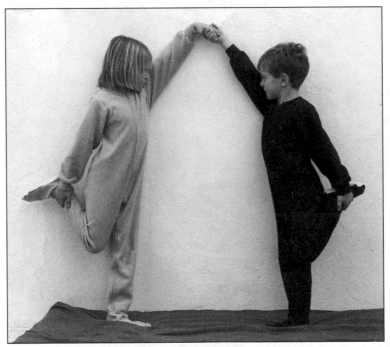

"Now, it's easy to balance and rest here for a long time."

" I feel like a sunflower growing up the wall."

Back-to-Back Dancers

BENEFITS: This pose opens the shoulder joints, expands the chest, balances the nervous system, enhances mental concentration and makes the back and legs supple.

Stand back-to-back with your partner, with your foot close to the wall. Inhaling, stretch your front arm up as straight as possible and hold your partner's hand. Exhaling, let the outside of your other arm and leg rest against the wall. This will help you keep your balance as you lift your leg that is next to the wall, bend the knee and hold your ankle with your hand.

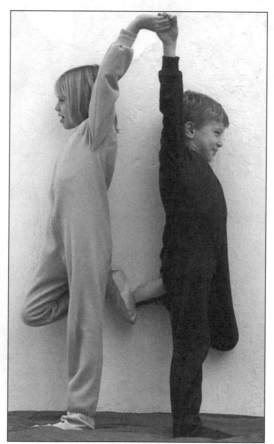

As you balance here, breathe down through your leg and into your foot. Imagine that you have roots that go deep into the earth.

Rest here as long as you like, then slowly release your arm and leg, reverse positions and try it with your other leg.

How does it feel?

"It feels easier to breathe deep into my chest."

"It feels like we're helping each other grow."

Double Cactus

BENEFITS: This deep three-part breathing is a classic Yoga breathing exercise known as the Yogic Breath. It expands breathing capacity, soothes the nervous system and is physically and emotionally nourishing. The reversed blood flow gives a rest to the heart and quiets the mind. It is very soothing for tired legs and has a calming effect on body, mind and spirit.

Lie with your hips against the wall and the backs of your legs touching the wall. Bend your arms at the elbows and bring your hands up to rest in the shape of a cactus with the palms of your hands facing the sky.

Breathe in deeply and feel the breath expand your tummy, as if you are blowing up a balloon. As you exhale, let your tummy deflate completely, as if all the air has gone out of the balloon.

On the next inhalation, your tummy expands first, and then your rib cage expands. Exhaling, your tummy deflates and then your rib cage does.

Again, breathe in deeply. First let your tummy expand, then your rib cage. Feel your chest expand and your chest bone rise. Exhale long, feeling your tummy deflate first, then your rib cage and finally your chest.

Continue like this for three deep breaths. Observe your tummy, rib cage and chest expand completely each time you breathe in, and deflate each time you breathe out.

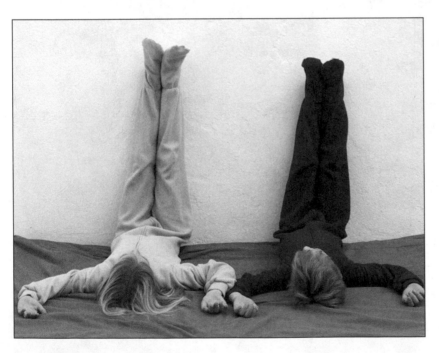

Double Cactus

Close your eyes and rest here as long as you like, enjoying this deep three-part breath as you observe your balloon growing bigger and then deflating with each breath.

How do you feel?

"I feel like my balloon is getting bigger and bigger with each breath."

"I feel as quiet as a cactus."

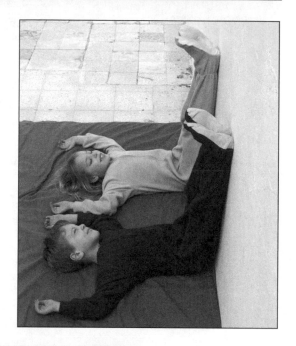

Resting Cactus

When you are ready to release the Cactus Pose, slowly roll down and rest on your side for a few minutes.

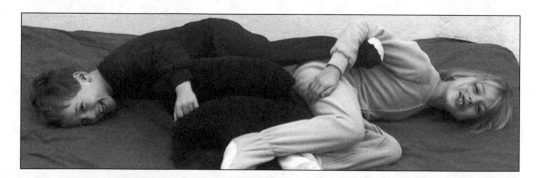

Tête-à-Tête

Benefits: This calming pose prepares both body and mind for a restful sleep.

Sit on your knees facing your partner and fall forward to bring your forehead to rest on the mat. Slowly, scoot toward your partner until the top of your heads touch. Rest your arms on the mat alongside your body, with the palms of your hands facing the sky.

As you exhale long and slowly, let all your muscles relax and feel your body melting into the mat. Feel the tops of your feet, your legs, and knees growing softer and sinking into the mat. Let your shoulders expand from side to side and feel your chest and tummy relax more, until your muscles are so relaxed that you don't want to move.

As you inhale, imagine the breath coming in the top of your head and expanding all the way down your spine. Now hold the breath in for a moment and concentrate on your tailbone at the base of your spine. Feel like you have a tail that is so heavy that it makes your hips sit down more toward your feet. Exhale, letting your breath soften all your muscles and joints even more.

Rest here as long as you like, enjoying this state of stillness.

How do you feel?

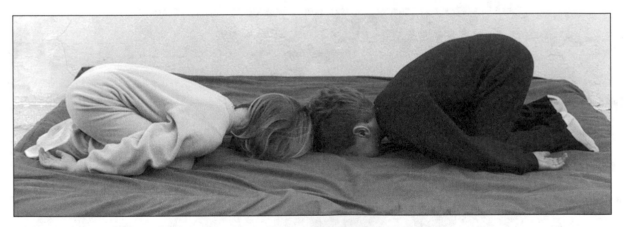

"I feel as silent as a mouse."
"We'll have sweet dreams tonight."

Meditation

Sit in a comfortable position with your legs crossed. Rest the backs of your hands on your knees and gently bring your thumb and index fingers together.

Close your eyes and breathe in deeply. Visualize the breath coming in the top of your head and expanding all the way down your spine. Now concentrate on your tailbone for a few moments. On the exhalation, picture your breath expanding back up through each vertebra of your spine and out the top of your head.

Continue like this for three breaths. With each exhalation, let the breath become softer and slower. Now, begin to concentrate on the space between each breath. Inhale deeply, then concentrate on the space before the exhalation. Exhale long, and concentrate on the silent space before the inhalation. Continue like this, sinking deeper and deeper into the silent space between each breath. Rest here as long as you like, enjoying this deep silence.

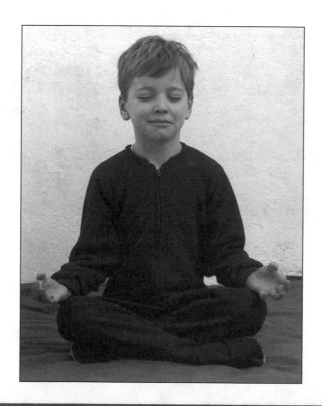

Contemplation

Concentrate on the
moment when you fall
asleep, the moment when
you slip from wakefulness
to slumber.

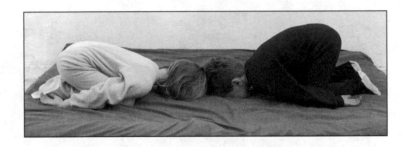

There is no thought, no
work, no worry. Rest here
a few moments enjoying
this state of stillness.

Sweet Dreams

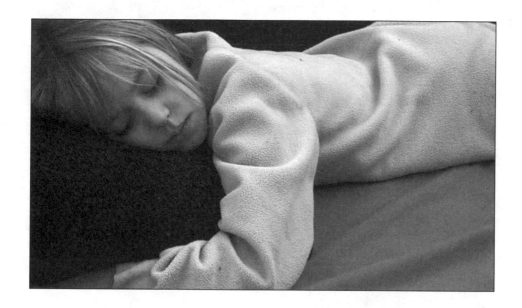

"I'm dreaming of a friendly laughing cobra who is gliding up a tall steeple to teach the whole world to be happy and kind."

Photo Credits

Chapter	Models	Photographer
1	Khadija and Youssef Rull Boussen La Marsa, Tunisia	Wes Gerrish
2	Katherine and Andrew Scrimgeour Aberdeen, Scotland	Wes Gerrish
3	Elspeth and Lucie Vovk Ayr, Scotland	Teressa Asencia
	Mary and Emily Byrne Dublin, Ireland	Teressa Asencia
	Sylvia and Katherine Scrimgeour Aberdeen, Scotland	Wes Gerrish
	Annick and Shann Liegl Laudun, France	Wes Gerrish
	Lee Li Chiao and Angel Lee Shanghai, China	Cheng Kun Lin
4	Annick, Darwin and Shann Liegl Laudun, France	Wes Gerrish
5	Jean-Claude Robeul and Siena Bevan Uzès, France	Wes Gerrish
	Susan Nachman Laguna Beach, CA, US	Joshua Nachman
	Shoshana Nachman Baltimore, MD, US	Tracy Bennett
6	Khadija and Youssef Rull Boussen La Marsa, Tunisia	Wes Gerrish

About the Author

Teressa Asencia has taught Yoga for twenty–five years in California, New York, Montreal, China, Tunisia and France. She has written and produced several Yoga videos and three Yoga television series. Her TV series *Welcome to Hatha Yoga* was shown daily on CBC TV in Canada; her *Yoga for Stress* series was shown on the Women's Network across Canada daily and aired on many PBS stations in the US.

She has danced and taught creative dance for many years. Currently, she dances Bharata Natyam, classical East Indian dance. Her award–winning documentary, "A Dance the Gods Yearn to Witness," depicts the rich history and tradition of Bharata Natyam.

Teressa lives in the south of France and teaches Yoga workshops internationally.